Contents

Foreword

First aid is never a substitute for medical help, but a means by which the informed layman can take lifesaving measures in emergencies, and avoid doing harm, before the doctor comes. This book is designed to give you quick step-by-step instructions in what to do first when emergencies strike.

The first-aid measures described are up to date and reflect current concepts and practices. The book was prepared and reviewed in consultation with eminent authorities, and the editors feel fortunate in having had the services of Donald G. Cooley, a long-time contributor to *Better Homes & Gardens* who is well known for his books and articles on medical subjects, in preparation of the text.

We urge that you familiarize yourself with the contents of the book *before* emergencies arise, so you will be prepared to take immediate action to avert tragedy. Keep the book always in the same place—such as the family medicine cabinet—so that it is immediately available when every second counts. Ideally, another copy should be in your home-away-from-home—the family automobile. At least one member of the family should take a first-aid course, such as the training given by the Red Cross.

The Editors

Better Homes & Gardens

Better Homes & Gardens

First aid

for your family

First rules for first aid

Take these steps in serious emergencies

If patient has stopped breathing:

Give immediate *mouth to mouth resuscitation* (see page 10).

Make sure that *air passages are open* in *any* unconscious or injured patient. Turn head to one side if nose and mouth are filled with fluid, blood, vomit. Wipe out with finger or handkerchief. Pull tongue forward if it has slipped back to plug throat.

If bleeding is serious:

Apply *pressure* directly over wound until bleeding stops.

Press *hard* with your hand against gauze, wadded cloth, clean handkerchief placed over wound. Use heel of bare hand in emergency. Keep pressing steadily; do not dab. If wound is in leg or arm, elevate limb above level of body and support with pillow or padding. *Do not* elevate injured part if bones are broken.

Do *not* apply tourniquet unless all other measures to stop bleeding fail (see *tourniquet*, page 24).

Prevent shock

Cover patient, keep him *comfortably* warm, not hot or sweaty.

If he can swallow, give warm fluids or "shock solution"—1 teaspoonful of salt, ½ teaspoon of baking soda, dissolved in 1 quart of water. Give by spoonful.

Do *not* give anything by mouth if patient is unconscious, half-conscious, vomiting, or if he has an abdominal wound.

Do not move victim

Never move patient from scene of accident while waiting for medical help, unless absolutely necessary. Keep him lying flat on back on level surface. Do not lift head, do not help him to sit or stand, do not bundle him into sitting position in back seat of car. Splinting should be done at the site of the accident. See *Transporting the injured* (page 46).

Summon doctor but first give resuscitation, if necessary; clear air passages; stop bleeding—seconds may save a life!

What you need to have on hand

Home First-aid Supplies (can be bought as unit at drugstore) should be kept in a special container or shelf, separate from other home medical supplies, should not contain poisons, and should never be locked with a key!

Always keep supplies in same place and return materials after use. Replace missing or depleted items promptly. Check condition of supplies regularly. If sterile packages have been broken, replace with fresh units.

Basic supplies below will suffice for immediate care of most injuries. You may add other items, but don't clutter the first-aid kit —essentials first!

Home first-aid supplies

For injuries

Sterile gauze compresses and pads, individually packaged, 2, 3, and 4 inches square

Sealed roller gauze bandages, 1, 2, and 3 inches wide (elastic crepe bandages are easiest to apply)

Clean sheets, pillowcases, handkerchiefs can be made relatively sterile by ironing just before use

Adhesive strip bandages with gauze pads, assorted sizes

Adhesive tape

Sterile absorbent cotton

Large triangular bandages: laundered and ironed muslin,

sheeting, about 40 inches square, cut diagonally to make 2 bandages

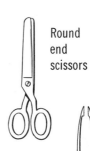

Round end scissors

Equipment

Scissors, rounded ends
Tweezers
Card of safety pins

Medicines and materials

Tube of petroleum jelly or package of impregnated gauze
Table salt (or salt tablets)
Baking soda
Aromatic spirits of ammonia (stimulant; dose: ½ teaspoonful in ½ glass of water).
Mineral or olive oil ("sweet oil"), sterile
Universal antidote for poisons (buy from druggist)

Flat end tweezers

Auto first-aid kit

Road accidents may cause injuries too large to be covered by a small gauze compress.

Large bandages may be needed for slings, burns, splinting. Improvised materials may not be available at the roadside. Carry these essentials in car in metal or plastic box, or impervious plastic bag. Antiseptics are not necessary if victim will soon receive medical care.

6 sterile gauze compresses or pads about 6 inches square
Sealed gauze compresses in smaller sizes

what you need to have on hand

3 or more rolls of sterile gauze bandages, 2-inch width and wider

6 or more triangular bandages (see *home first-aid supplies*)

Absorbent cotton

Petroleum jelly, tube

Scissors

Safety pins

Travelers' medical supplies

If you plan to travel in foreign countries, or to camp or work in regions remote from a doctor or hospital, ask your physician about medical supplies you should carry with you. Thermometers used in foreign countries are usually marked in the centigrade scale unfamiliar to most Americans. You may wish to take along a familiar Fahrenheit thermometer.

Home medicine cabinet

Common household remedies, as well as drugs prescribed by a physician, should be stored separately from tooth paste, shaving cream, and other simple items of daily use. Even the simple home

Important → medicines which are quite harmless if properly used may be toxic if taken in huge overdosage. If there are children around the house, home medicines should be kept under lock and key in a cabinet of their own, or at least should be dependably inaccessible to youngsters. In addition to first-aid supplies and medicines for personal use, the following items are useful to have on hand in readiness for emergency:

Clinical thermometers, oral and rectal

Ice bag

Hot water bottle

Eyecup

Paper cups

Flashlight

Tongue depressors

Cotton-tipped applicators

Rubbing alcohol

Milk of magnesia

Calamine lotion

For a safe medicine cabinet:

Do not take medicine in the dark or without reading label—if label is lost, discard bottle. . . . Throw out all prescription drugs left over from past illnesses. . . . Give a prescription drug only to the patient for whom the physician ordered it. . . . Date all drug supplies when you buy them. . . . Mark all poisons; seal lid with tape, run pin through cork, put sandpaper strip on bottle. . . . Dispose of old drugs safely—best done by pouring down sink—so children and pets can't get at them.

Mark poisons for quick identification

Big label

POISON

Pin through cork

Sandpaper strip

Artificial respiration

Important →

Examine immediately the breathing of any accident victim

If a person has stopped breathing *from any cause*, start artificial respiration at once. Seconds count! The most efficient and practical way to save a life is to blow your breath into the victim's lungs— like inflating a balloon, letting out the pressure, inflating again. You can do this without help or equipment. A child can save the life of an adult with this method.

Mouth to mouth (or mouth to nose) resuscitation

1. Tilt victim's head back so chin points upward.

2. Pull or push the jaw into a jutting-out position.

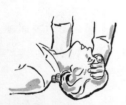

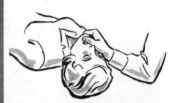

3.

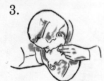

Open your mouth wide, place it tightly over the victim's mouth. Pinch victim's nostrils shut.

↑

Or close nostrils with the pressure of your cheek.
↓

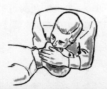

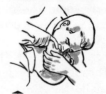

↑
Or close the victim's mouth and place your mouth over the nose.

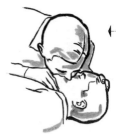

4.

← Blow into the victim's mouth or nose.

Remove your mouth, → turn your head to the side, listen for return outflow of air from victim's lungs.

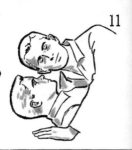

If foreign matter is visible in the victim's mouth, wipe it out quickly with your fingers or cloth wrapped around your fingers.

For an adult, blow vigorously at a rate of about 12 breaths per minute. For a child, take relatively shallow breaths at a rate of about 20 per minute.

If you are not getting air exchange (expansion of victim's chest, return outflow when you remove your mouth), recheck head and jaw positions; make sure mouth and throat are clear —Figures 1 and 2.

If you still do not get air exchange, turn victim on his side and give several sharp blows between shoulder blades in hope of dislodging foreign matter. Again sweep fingers through mouth to remove foreign matter. A handkerchief or cloth may be placed over the victim's mouth or nose if the rescuer wishes to avoid direct contact. Several layers of cloth will not greatly affect air exchange.

Start artificial respiration immediately and continue until doctor arrives or you are positive life is gone. It is the victim's only hope of life while rescuers with equipment are on the way.

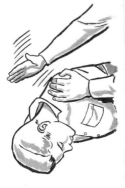

Several sharp pats between shoulder blades may dislodge foreign matter from victim's throat

artificial respiration

*Infants and small children
Mouth to mouth technique*

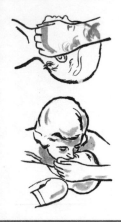

1. Clean visible foreign matter from mouth with finger; place child on back; use fingers of both hands to lift lower jaw from beneath and behind so it juts out (as with adults).

Place your mouth over *both mouth and nose* of child to make "leakproof" seal. Breathe into child with shallow puffs of air, about 20 per minute.

If air exchange seems to be blocked, and you cannot breathe easily into child, check "jutting out" position of jaw to be sure tongue has not fallen back and that airway is open.

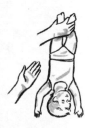

2. *If* air passages are still blocked, suspend child by ankles—or— hold child head-down over one of your arms and give several sharp pats between shoulder blades to help dislodge obstructing matter.

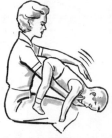

Continue artificial respiration until the victim begins to breathe for himself or until a physician pronounces the victim dead. Time your efforts to breathe into the victim to coincide with the victim's first attempt to breathe for himself.

Normally, recovery is rapid except in *electric shock*, and *drug* or *carbon monoxide* poisoning, which may require artificial respiration for long periods.

An **airway tube** *is* *desirable first-aid equipment*

Drugstores sell inexpensive "resuscitation tubes" made of plastic. One end is inserted over the victim's tongue, the other end projects and serves as a mouthpiece through which the rescuer breathes into the victim. Direct oral contact is avoided. The tubes come in child and adult sizes and are very desirable pieces of first-aid equipment to carry in a car and have in the home for emergencies. Follow directions for use of the tube very carefully or you may do more harm than good. If tube is not instantly available, give direct mouth to mouth respiration immediately.

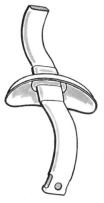

A resuscitation tube and the mouth to mouth technique are equally effective means of artificial respiration

Back pressure– arm lift *resuscitation*

Other resuscitation measures do not move so much air as direct mouth to mouth, are less efficient, more exhausting to the rescuer, but first-aiders should have an alternative, such as the Back Pressure-Arm Lift method. Wipe visible foreign matter from victim's mouth with finger or cloth wrapped around finger.
1. Place victim face down, bend his elbows, place his hands one

This method can be used only if victim has no arm injury

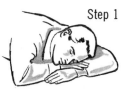

Step 1

artificial respiration

Step 2

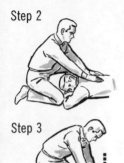

Step 3

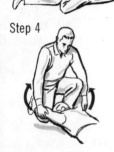

Step 4

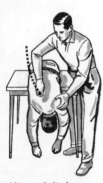

upon the other. Turn his head to one side, extend as far as possible so chin juts out.

2. Kneel at victim's head. Place your hands on flat of his back so your palms lie just below an imaginary line between his armpits.

3. Rock forward until your arms are nearly vertical, with weight of upper part of your body exerting steady even pressure downward on your hands.

4. Immediately draw the victim's arms up and toward you. Lift enough to feel resistance and tension at his shoulders. Then lower his arms to ground. Repeat about 12 times per minute. Check mouth frequently for obstruction.

A Chest Pressure-Arm Lift method is also taught by the Red Cross. Check with your local unit.

Choking *from foreign object in windpipe or throat*

If a child, hold up by heels and slap back hard between shoulder blades. If an adult, have him lie face down over edge of bed or table, head and shoulders hanging down. Slap back hard between shoulder blades.

If object is not dislodged, rush to hospital. Do not try to grasp object with your fingers unless you can obviously hook your fingers around it. There is great danger of pushing object farther down throat. If breathing stops, start *artificial respiration* at once.

If an adult, have him lie over table edge; slap between shoulder blades

Drowning

Begin *artificial respiration* the instant a near-drowned person is landed. Do not waste time trying to "empty water out of the lungs" by jackknifing or rolling on a barrel. Turn victim's head to side, clean foreign material from mouth, so stomach contents can clear. Begin artificial respiration. ← Important Continue without interruption until help comes. Check to see that tongue is clear and airway open at all times. Keep victim warm.

← Important
Keep victim's tongue
out of throat; keep
air passages open
at all times

Gas poisoning
Carbon monoxide poisoning

Get victim into fresh air. Protect *yourself* in entering gas-filled area. A wet cloth over your nose does not protect you. Tie a rope around yourself so someone can pull you out if you fall.

If the victim's breathing has stopped or is irregular, give artificial respiration continuously. Send for oxygen device from local police, fire department, or ambulance service. Give continuous ← Important artificial respiration until trained operator with oxygen arrives.

Prevent asphyxiation tragedies

. . . Children put small objects into their mouths and sometimes "inhale" them. Keep beans, peanuts, fruit pits, pins, buttons, beads, coins out of reach of small

artificial respiration

children. Permit no toy smaller than child's fist. Check toys for parts such as doll's eyes that may come loose and be taken into the windpipe. . . . Never leave a small child alone in a bathtub for a second. . . . Have gas heaters, ranges, appliances, home furnaces checked regularly by trained service men. Never run car engine with garage door closed. Have car exhaust system checked periodically.

Electric shock

First, shut off current or remove victim from contact (extreme caution—see directions)
then give immediate prolonged artificial respiration until help comes

Serious electric shock paralyzes breathing centers, causes unconsciousness. Ordinary house current can cause fatal shock under some circumstances.

Don't touch victim until current is turned off or victim is free of contact with current—you may be electrocuted yourself.

If indoors, or if switch is near, turn off current at switch.

If outdoors (live wires, no switch) have someone phone electric company to turn off current, but don't wait for this. If victim's muscular contractions have thrown him free of current he may be touched at once. Otherwise, proceed with *extreme caution*.

Important → *Insulate yourself* from the earth and the victim with *dry* nonconducting materials, such as a long length of dry rope or cloth. But remember that very few materials are bone-dry, and that you are risking your life.

Never use anything metallic, wet, or damp

It may be simplest to pull wire away from victim, as below:

Stand on *dry* newspapers, *dry* board, *dry* rubber floor mat of car, *dry* folded coat.

Use *dry* stick, *dry* board, *dry* rolled newspapers or floor mat to pull or push wire from contact with victim.

If victim lies on wire he may be pushed from it with a *dry* board. Or he may be pulled away with a *dry* rope. Insulate your hands with *dry* gloves, cloth, newspapers. If your hand is insulated you may with *caution* grasp a *dry* part of the patient's clothing and drag him away (do not touch shoes; nails may conduct).

After contact is broken, give immediate *artificial respiration* and continue until help arrives. If victim's body stiffened, do not assume that he cannot be revived. Breathing centers paralyzed by electric shock take a long time to recover—victims have recovered after eight hours of artificial respiration. Don't give up.

Lightning

Use the same first aid as for electric shock except that victims may be touched immediately and artificial respiration can begin at once.

To avoid danger from lightning, seek lowest point, ditch, depres-

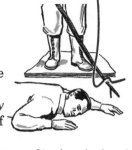

Stand on dry board or dry newspapers

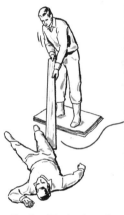

Push with dry board or stick to free victim from wire

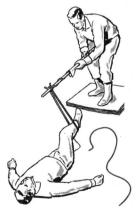

Use dry rope to pull arm or leg from wire

artificial respiration

sion; avoid isolated trees. One of safest places to be in a lightning storm is inside a car.

Prevent electrocution accidents

. . . Have all switches and appliances in locations that can't be touched from bath, shower, sink. . . . Never have electrical appliances where they can fall into water, tub, sink. . . . Don't touch anything electrical while standing on wet floors or in puddles. . . . Touch nothing electrical if your hands are wet. . . . Have electrical equipment permanently grounded. . . . Remove fuse before making electrical repairs. . . . Replace all frayed electric cords. Children chewing on frayed wires can get frightful mouth burns or fatal shock. Cover unused wall sockets with protective plates, seal with adhesive tape, or use inexpensive blank plugs, so children can't push nails or hairpins into openings and receive serious or fatal shock. . . . Never touch a dangling wire; may be charged by crossing power line farther back. Call utility company if wire is down in yard; keep children away. . . . Don't use metal ladders in proximity to electricity (may be grounded if touch live wires—short circuits). . . . If car runs into live wire, touch no metal, stay in car until help arrives.

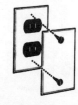

Cover all unused wall sockets with protective plates

Bleeding

Serious, from wounds, injuries

Remove enough clothing to see wound clearly. Cover wound with sterile compress and apply *firm hand pressure* directly over wound. Exert firm, steady pressure, not intermittent. Press with finger, hand, or heel of hand until bleeding stops.

Use clean materials, such as sterile gauze, folded clean handkerchiefs, freshly laundered or ironed towels, strips from sheets to cover bleeding point.

If no sterile items are available, do not hesitate to use clothing, soiled materials, or bare hand to stanch flow of blood by pressure. Blood loss is more dangerous than immediate risk of infection.

Deep cuts

Severed blood vessels

Spurting or oozing blood

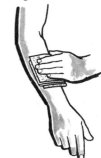

Press clean cloth firmly against wound

Bleeding from **legs, arms**

If wound is in arm or leg, *elevate* limb, support with pillows or similar padding. Raise bleeding part above level of body. *Do not* elevate limb if bones are broken or fracture is suspected.

Think first of pressure in severe bleeding wound. Direct finger or hand pressure is the safest and most rapid measure to stop bleeding. Pressure and elevation of limb will control most bleeding.

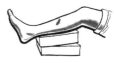

Raise bleeding arm or leg above level of body, if no fracture is suspected

bleeding

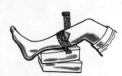

Bandage must not be too tight; wound area may swell

Pressure dressing

When bleeding stops, apply *pressure dressing*. Put gauze compress or folded layers of clean cloth over bleeding point (do not use fluffy absorbent cotton in direct contact with wound). Press compress with fingers and apply suitable bandage to fix dressing in place. Preferably, use gauze compress bandage: strip of cloth with thick layer of gauze in center and tails Important →for wrapping and tying. Many bleeding wounds can be controlled by *pressure dressings alone*.

Bandage must not be *too tight*. Wound area may swell. Inspect occasionally. If edge of bandage cuts into flesh it is too tight; loosen. Otherwise, do not disturb or remove bandage after it is applied. If blood oozes into bandage, cover with another layer of bandaging material.

General measures

Do *not* apply salves, ointments, or any medicines to deep wounds, unless told to by doctor. Covering wound with sterile gauze or clean cloth protects against further contamination.

Do *not* try to cleanse a deep or seriously bleeding wound (bleeding cleanses it internally) unless medical help is long delayed or there is gross contamination.

If essential, cleanse skin around wound with clean (tap or boiled)

Contaminated wound may be cleansed with soapsuds, if not bleeding badly

water stirred with soap to make sudsy solution. Scrub your hands first with soap and water.

Cover wound and small area of surrounding skin with sterile gauze. Dip a tuft of sterile absorbent cotton into soapy solution, apply gently to exposed skin, stroking *away* from wound.

Use fresh cotton tuft for each stroke. Greases and oils may be removed by kerosene, naphtha, rubbing alcohol. Always wash *away* from wound. *Keep patient lying down.*

Suspect shock

Some degree of *shock* is imminent in all cases of serious bleeding. Cover patient, keep him comfortable, not overheated. Loosen tight clothing. Cut clothing away if necessary, to avoid twisting, turning, or manipulating patient. *If patient is conscious*, not vomiting, give saline mixture made by dissolving 1 teaspoonful of table salt and ½ teaspoonful of baking soda in 1 quart of water.

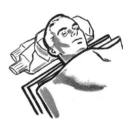

Have shock victim lie flat on back

Give in small sips as tolerated by patient. Do not give *stimulants*. Do not give anything by mouth if patient has *abdominal wound or if internal bleeding* is suspected.

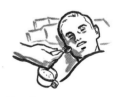

Give fluids only after bleeding has stopped

Pressure points
to stop bleeding

In all serious bleeding, *first* try *manual pressure* directly upon

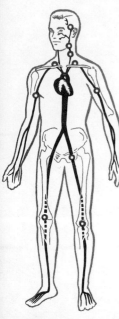

Points to press if
bandage does not
stop bleeding

wound, *pressure bandage*, and *elevation of limb*.

These are most *rapid* and *safe* measures which control most cases of serious bleeding and need no special training. If bleeding does not stop, or resumes after pressure bandage is applied, press with fingers or hand against proper *pressure point of body where blood vessels pass over bone*.

Pressure at these points shuts off blood like clamping a rubber hose. But *do not waste time* in a serious emergency trying to locate pressure points unless you know about them from first-aid training (ask your Red Cross chapter about instruction courses).

If *immediate* application of pressure against compress directly over wound does not stop violent flow of blood, or if bleeding resumes, exert finger or hand pressure at these points:

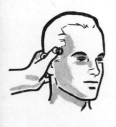

Bleeding from head above eye level

Press with finger against head just in front of the ear.

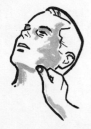

Bleeding below eye and above jawbone

Press fingers against notch in jawbone which is about one inch in front of the angle of the jaw.

Bleeding from neck, mouth, throat

Place thumb against back of neck, fingers on side of neck below Adam's apple in depression at side of windpipe (*not over* windpipe). Press fingers *toward* thumb.

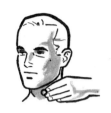

Bleeding from armpit, shoulder, upper arm

Place fingers or thumb in hollow behind patient's collarbone, press against upper surface of first rib.

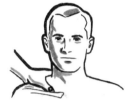

Bleeding from hand, forearm, lower two-thirds of arm

Press against arm bone halfway between armpit and elbow, thumb inside arm, fingers outside.

Bleeding from palm of hand: Place thick pad covered with sterile gauze in palm, close fingers over it, bandage into closed fist.

Forearm bleeding: Pressure pad inside elbow, tighten forearm against pad, bind.

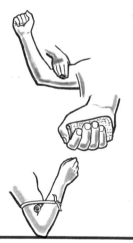

Bleeding from foot, leg, thigh

Place heel of hand in middle of depression on inner side of thigh, just below fold of groin, press down against bone.

Bleeding below knee: Pressure pad in back of knee, tighten lower leg against pad, bind.

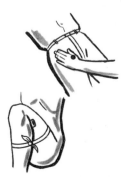

bleeding

Tourniquet
for life-threatening bleeding

Important → *A tourniquet is a dangerous instrument.* It is a constricting band around a limb which shuts off blood to points beyond it. Tissues die (gangrene) if deprived of blood too long.

A tourniquet is of value as a first-aid tool *only when there is partial or complete amputation of a body part*—at risk of a limb to save a life. There must always be unbroken skin between the wound and the tourniquet.

Massive bleeding
from **arm** *or* **leg**

General *position* of tourniquet:
   Between wound and heart.
   For *arm* bleeding: about hand's width below armpit.
   For *leg* or *thigh* bleeding: about a hand's width below groin.
   Place tourniquet as close to wound as possible (to save more of limb if amputation becomes necessary) but not at edge or directly over wound.

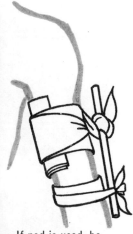

If pad is used, be sure it is over the artery

Tourniquet materials

Any fairly wide band (about 2 inches) long enough to go twice around limb with ends left for tying. Belt, stocking, scarf, strip torn from clothing or cut from inner tube in emergency—many first-aid kits contain tourniquet that buckles. Do *not* use wire, rope, cord, which cut into flesh, except in dire emergency.

How to apply tourniquet

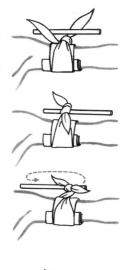

Wrap band twice around limb, tie half knot, place stick over knot, tie tight knot over stick. Twist stick to tighten *just enough to stop blood flow.* Tie free end of tightened stick with another bandage to hold in position.

Do not loosen or remove tourniquet once it has been carefully applied. Fatal blood loss may result from intermittent loosening. Get as soon as possible to doctor who can remove tourniquet and replace blood loss.

Leave tourniquet in plain sight. *Do not hide* with bandage, clothing. Mark *"TK"* on patient's forehead with lipstick, charred match end. Note *time* when tourniquet was applied.

Internal bleeding

Injuries may cause *internal* bleeding, with or without outward signs of blood loss. *Suspect* internal bleeding after any severe blow, blunt or crushing injury to abdomen, chest, torso.

Some signs of internal bleeding:

From *stomach:* vomited material looks like large coffee grounds.

From *upper intestines:* stools contain dark tarry material (partly digested blood).

bleeding

Important
Prompt medical care
is urgent for
internal bleeding

Do not give
stimulants

Important →

From *lower intestines:* bright red blood in stools.

From *chest, lungs:* coughed-up blood is bright red, frothy.

Some injuries give only *general* signs of internal hemorrhage: *restlessness, anxiety, thirst, pallor, weakness, rapid but weak pulse.* Suspect internal bleeding; get doctor at once.

Keep patient warm, quiet, lying on back, head turned to one side if vomiting or coughing. Keep breathing passages clear of obstruction. Patient with bleeding from lung may not be able to breathe if lying flat—if so, prop high enough so he can breathe.

Nosebleed

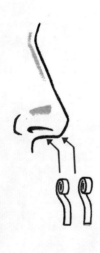

Quickest way to stop nosebleeds: Pinch nose between thumb and forefinger for 10 or 15 minutes.

Another way: Put pad of cotton, tissue, or soft cloth under upper lip. Press against nose firmly with forefinger laid along lip.

If bleeding persists, plug nostril *gently* with small strip of loosely rolled gauze. Push backward (*not* upward) into nostril no farther than little finger can push it. Leave strip of gauze dangling for easy removal.

Do not blow nose for several hours after bleeding has stopped. Most nosebleeds stop by themselves and are not serious. If nosebleeding persists or recurs, see doctor.

Shock

Every serious accident, burn, poisoning, injury is virtually always accompanied by some degree of *shock*, perhaps mild, but often serious, and fatal if shock becomes irreversible. Shock is caused by bodily reactions which slow or stop the circulatory mechanisms, and symptoms are essentially those of insufficient blood supply to vital organs.

← Important

After giving immediate lifesaving first aid—stopping bleeding, making sure patient's breathing passageways are open, giving artificial resuscitation if necessary—always think of shock before taking other time-consuming first-aid steps. *Expect* shock to develop after any serious injury. Take preventive steps *before* the doctor arrives to take over.

Give treatment for shock after any serious injury; do not wait for symptoms to appear

Signs of shock

Weakness
Rapid but weak pulse
Pale face
Skin cold, clammy with perspiration of forehead, palms; patient may have chills
Thirst
Nausea
Shallow, irregular breathing
Blood pressure very low (late sign)

shock

Immediate first aid to lessen shock

First deal with any immediate life-threatening emergency that the injury requires.

1. Have patient lie flat, head level with or lower than rest of body (unless he has head injury, in which case, elevate head slightly. Caution: see *broken neck*).

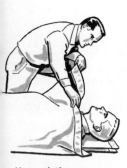

Elevate legs 12 to 18 inches above head, if nature of injury permits

Equivalent of head-lowering, to help flow of blood to heart and brain, is most easily accomplished by elevating legs to height of 12 to 18 inches, if nature of injury permits.

2. Cover patient, protect him from cold ground, air, loss of body heat. Keep him warm but not too warm—just on the warm side of chilling. Object is not to heat the patient but to keep him from cooling.

3. Do not let patient see injury. Reassure him. Handle very gently. Pain increases shock.

Keep victim warm but do not cause sweating

4. If patient is conscious, not vomiting, does not have abdominal injury, give *shock solution*: 1 teaspoonful of table salt, ½ teaspoonful of baking soda, dissolved in 1 quart of water. Measure proportions carefully.

Give patient all he will drink.

If available, a cup of strong black coffee or tea is helpful.

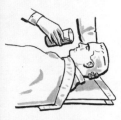

Give shock solution or water that is not hot or cold

Get doctor as soon as possible. Patient should be in better condition when doctor arrives if you take above steps promptly.

Broken bones

Falls, car crashes, crushing injuries, or blows may break bones (cause fractures). A *simple* fracture exists under unbroken skin and may not be obvious. A *compound* fracture shows bone protruding from the skin, or an open wound at the fracture site; frequently there is severe bleeding.

Suspect broken bones if: ← Signs of broken bones
Victim can't move injured part
Part is deformed, wrong shape
Pain when trying to move
Lack of feeling when touched
Swelling and blueness of skin
If in doubt, treat as a fracture.

General principles of first aid for fractures

Great harm can be done if patient is moved hastily, pulled, bundled into back seat of car, allowed to stand, sit up, or move injured part. A fracture itself almost never is an emergency that requires great speed in treatment. Unless essential for safety, *do not move* or ← Important disturb patient while waiting for doctor or ambulance.

If victim *must* be moved from great danger, pull at legs or armpits along long axis of body.

Examine first for other injuries.

broken bones

Stop serious bleeding by hand pressure on gauze dressing over wound.

Check mouth, throat for possible obstruction of breathing. Keep airway open. Give artificial respiration if needed.

If necessary, cut away clothing with great care not to disturb injured part.

Keep patient warm, lying down.

Do not put pillow under head if neck is injured but block head with padding to prevent neck movement.

If medical help will be delayed and patient must be transported:

Do not try to set bones.

Always apply *splints* before moving or transporting patient.

Splint the patient where he lies.

Apply clean dressing and bandage (no antiseptic) if bone protrudes through skin or skin is broken.

See *Transporting the injured*.

Splinting materials

The purpose of a splint is to give the broken part constant support, immobilize it, prevent bone ends from grinding together. Almost anything that is rigid enough will serve in an emergency—boards, sticks, rifle barrel, umbrella, cane, jack handle, tightly rolled magazine or floor mat. The splint must be long enough to extend above and below adjacent joints to prevent motion. Hard objects must

Use almost any rigid material to make an emergency splint

be well *padded* with cotton, cloth, soft materials, before placing in contact with injured part.

Broken arms or legs
Forearm or wrist

Have patient lie on back. *Gently* place forearm across chest, right angle to upper arm, palm flat on chest. Prepare 2 padded splints: an inside splint from elbow to palm, an outside splint from elbow to back of fingers. Tie splint in place with 2 bandages, one above, one below the fracture. Adjust necktie sling to hold finger tips 3 or 4 inches above level of elbow unless forearm is more comfortable at a different level.

Newspaper splint: cover fracture site with thick gauze bandage, roll folded newspaper over it; tie.

Upper arm
(elbow to shoulder)

Place arm gently at side in as natural position as possible, forearm at right angles lying across chest, palm side in. Place 1 padded splint outside arm, from slightly below elbow to slightly above shoulder. Tie with two cloth strips, one above, one below fracture site. Support forearm with necktie sling. Bandage upper arm to body with towel or cloth passed around splint and chest, tied under opposite arm.

If splint unavailable, bind arm

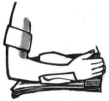

Newspaper for emergency wrist splint

Tie splint above and below fracture

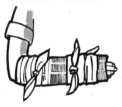

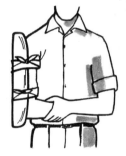

Make splint longer than bone it supports

If fingers turn blue, loosen splint

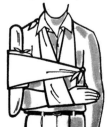

broken bones

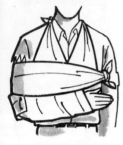

Do not straighten or bend broken elbow

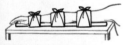

Tie splint to upper arm and forearm, but not to elbow

Pull foot slowly to straighten leg into normal position

firmly to side with cloth strips around chest. Support with sling.

In arm fractures: Watch patient's finger tips. If they become blue or swollen, loosen splint slightly. Remove rings, bracelets, wrist watches, which would be hard to get off should arm and fingers swell.

Elbow

If elbow is bent, *do not* try to straighten it. Put arm in sling and bind it firmly to body.

If arm and elbow are straight, leave that way. Put a single padded splint on inside of the arm, from finger tips nearly to the armpit. Tie securely above and below (not over) the elbow. Caution: Splint must not protrude into armpit with such force as to cut off blood supply.

Broken leg (lower leg, knee to ankle)

Caution! Jagged bones may break through skin or cut blood vessels if roughly handled. Use care.

Remove shoe gently; cut laces, leather. Grasp foot firmly and pull slowly to straighten leg and foot to normal position. If working alone, tie feet together after leg is in normal position. Otherwise, hold leg in position while assistant prepares splints.

Pillow splint: Slide folded blanket, robe, or firm pillow under injured leg—lift leg no more than necessary, while supporting broken bones. Tie pillow splint around leg in five places. Use stick or any rigid object for added stiffness.

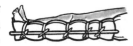

Lift leg no more than necessary while applying splint

Board splints: Two padded splints, boards about 4 inches high, reaching from just above knee to just beyond heel. Pad especially well at ankle. Put a splint on each side of leg; tie as shown.

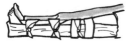

Pad board splints well at ankles

If no splints available, put blanket, folded towels, soft cloth between patient's legs and tie injured leg to sound leg (but *not* if break is near ankle).

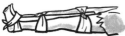

If splints unavailable, tie legs together

Broken thigh
(upper leg, hip)

Very serious. Treat for shock. Get doctor as soon as possible. Injured leg may be shortened, foot flops, victim can't raise heel from ground when lying with knees flat. But there may be no deformity, injury may look like a bruise. When in doubt, treat as fracture. Put one hand under heel, other over instep, steady the limb and pull gently into normal position. If working alone, tie feet together temporarily.

Treat for shock; get medical help; gently straighten leg

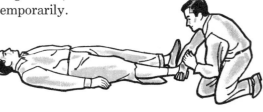

Prepare 7 broad long bandages or cloth strips. Use small stick to push them under hollows beneath knees and back, work into positions as shown.

Push bandages under body and injured leg with a small stick

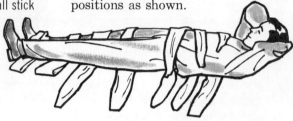

Use two board splints, 4 to 6 inches wide, well padded. Outer splint should reach from armpit to heel, inner splint from crotch to heel. Tie as shown.

Do not tie splint bandages too tightly

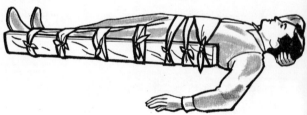

If no inner splint available, put padding between legs and tie legs together. If no splints available, pad well between legs to use un-injured leg as a splint.

If toes become bluish, swollen, loosen splint slightly.

Broken kneecap

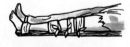

Apply splint from heel to buttocks for broken kneecap

Straighten leg gently, rest leg on 4-inch-wide board splint underneath leg. Pad splint, extra padding under knee and ankle. Tie as shown. Leave kneecap exposed. Watch for swelling; loosen ties if

.necessary. Caution: If knee joint fractured, or if you're in doubt, do not try to straighten leg.

Broken ankle

Pillow splint or rolled blanket extending well beyond heel. Tie as shown.

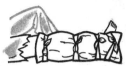

Tie pillow to ankle

Broken foot or toes

Place padded splint under sole of foot, tie as shown, snugly, but not too tightly.

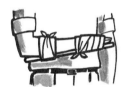

Padded foot-splint

Hand fractures

Padded splint under palm, from near elbow to beyond finger tips. Tie as shown.

Trunk fractures
Collarbone

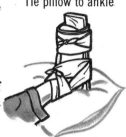

Splint under palm

Indications: Fractured ends usually can be felt by passing fingers over curved bone above top ribs. Patient usually cannot raise arm above shoulder. Injured shoulder lower than other when arms hang.

Pull shoulders back to lessen pain

Put arm in triangular bandage sling, finger tips exposed, adjust height to most comfortable position. Tie arm to body with towel or cloth over sling.

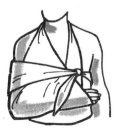

Ribs

Broken rib indications: Pain on breathing or coughing. Shallow

broken bones

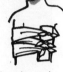

If bandages increase
chest pain, they
should be removed

If patient
coughs up blood →

breathing to lessen pain. Patient may hold hand over break to limit chest motion when he breathes. Put broad pad over break. Put broad cloth strip around chest, tie single knot over pad. Tighten second knot. Tie two similar bandages in place, as shown, to give firm support. Broken ribs should not be bandaged with great force and tightness because of danger of rib end puncturing lung.

Alternative: Make a tight chest binder from pillowcase, sheet strip, any large cloth. Wrap tightly around chest when patient exhales; fasten the chest binder securely with safety pins.

Caution! If patient coughs up bloody froth or bright red blood (lung puncture) *do not* apply tight bandages. Get medical aid immediately. Give first aid for *shock* until doctor takes over.

Pelvis

Serious! Broken bones of pelvis (basin-shaped structure between spine and lower limbs) may damage important organs. Car accidents, squeezing, crushing hip injuries may fracture pelvis. Signs: great pain in pelvic region; possible difficulty in urination. If in doubt, treat as fracture. Extreme care in handling!

Don't move patient if medical help is on way. Keep him lying down. Bandage ankles and knees together, legs straight or knees bent, whichever is most comfortable to patient.

If patient must be moved, slide broad bandage under hollow of back, work under hips, tie snugly but not tightly or fasten with safety pins. Transport face up on board or stretcher (see *Transporting the injured*).

Place broken pelvis victim flat on back

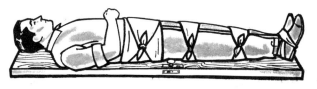

Head and face fractures
Jaw (lower)

Jaw usually sags; saliva trickles; teeth out of line or loosened; possible bleeding from mouth. Raise lower jaw gently to normal position, support with broad bandage under chin tied at top of head.

If patient vomits, bleeds from mouth, *remove* bandage at once. Turn head to side, support jaw gently with hand, replace bandage when vomiting stops.

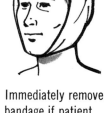

Immediately remove bandage if patient vomits or bleeds from the mouth

Nose

Don't splint a broken nose. Gauze may be inserted into nostrils if not forced in upward direction, but pushed gently straight back. If there is bleeding, press sides of nose together between thumb and index finger for several minutes. Press cold cloths over nose. Have

broken bones

Any serious blow
to head may cause
skull fracture; call
doctor at once and
give first aid

patient hold head back slightl breathe through mouth. Apply sterile dressing if open wound. Get prompt medical attention to prevent deformity.

Skull (Fracture, Concussion)

Assume that any severe blow to the head, whether or not the patient is "knocked out," is a skull fracture or concussion (bruise of the brain). *Any person who has suffered head injury should be kept quiet and be seen by a doctor as soon as possible*, even if he seems to have "recovered." Symptoms may be delayed.

Immediate First Aid: Keep patient lying down, warm; do not let him sit up or walk. Keeping quiet is the only first-aid means of reducing internal bleeding.

If face is *flushed*, raise head slightly with pillow or pad.

If face is *pale*, keep head on level with body or slightly lower.

Give *nothing* by mouth.

Turn head to side, so secretions can escape from mouth.

Apply cold cloths to head.

If scalp is bleeding, bandage gauze compress lightly in place— do *not* press hard on skull bruise or depressed area (may drive bone fragments into brain).

If necessary, transport in lying-down position, head supported by pads at sides to prevent any jarring.

Get doctor as soon as possible.

Broken neck or back

Utter tragedy can result if a victim of spinal injury is moved by well-intentioned but uninformed persons. Slight movement of head or back may sever nerves and cause permanent paralysis or death. What you *don't* do the first few minutes is more important than what you do:

DO NOT move or lift patient from where he lies until medical help arrives.

DO NOT bend or twist his head or body in any direction.

DO NOT put pillow under his head or give drink of water or a cigarette.

DO NOT pull him out if he is imprisoned in wrecked car, unless danger of fire—wait for medical help.

DO NOT jackknife him into back seat of a car and rush to hospital—first see *Transporting the injured.*

← DON'TS that may prevent tragedies

What to do:

Suspect broken back or neck and treat as fracture if patient has had bad fall, "whiplash" neck injury, crushing or impact injury, any accident in which back or neck is bent or struck.

    If patient is conscious, ask him to move hands and fingers. If he cannot, suspect neck fracture. If he cannot move feet and toes, suspect back fracture. He may complain of pain in neck or back.

A slight pain or discomfort may be the only symptom of broken neck or back

broken bones

There may be no other sign. Consider circumstances of injury.

Summon doctor and ambulance. While waiting for help, keep patient warm, covered, unmoving. Do not lift him or allow others to do so.

Important → If patient *must* be transported to medical aid, see *Transporting the injured*.

Prevent broken bones. Good housekeeping—nothing to fall down, to trip over; dry, clean floors. Carpet slippery floors; anchor small rugs by placing rubber sheet underneath. Good light everywhere; no dark cluttered stairways. Rubber mat in bathtub. Handrails where needed. Don't use furniture for stepladder. Position ladders securely; check rungs. Screen windows securely. Sprinkle icy walks with ashes or sand.

Bandages and bandaging

In an emergency, do not try to apply bandages in complex, precise, professional ways unless you have had special training. The first-aider's bandages will be replaced by a doctor. Elastic bandages, types which conform to body contours, adhesive compresses, help to make bandaging simpler.

1. First, apply sterile gauze compress big enough to cover wound. Apply bandage over compress.

2. Bind firmly but *not* too tightly—just enough pressure to stop flow of blood. Wound may swell and make bandage so tight as to shut off circulation. Watch for swelling, blueness, edge of bandage cutting into flesh—warnings to loosen bandage.

Materials

Sterile packaged materials in many sizes, including the largest, should be parts of every first-aid kit: roller gauze bandages (can be folded to make compresses), adhesive bandages, bandage compresses, sterile gauze compresses (get some large sizes), cotton rolls

Important
What Bandages Do:

Support body parts

Hold compresses in place

Help to stop bleeding

Protect wound from outside dirt

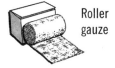

Roller gauze

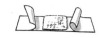

Adhesive compress

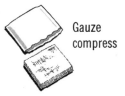

Gauze compress

Bandage compress

Absorbent cotton

Fold triangular bandage to make cravat

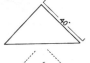

Universal dressing

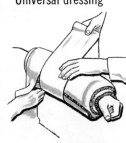

(never use fluffy cotton bandaged in direct contact with bleeding wound).

Freshly laundered and ironed sheets, handkerchiefs, napkins, pillowcases, towels make suitable improvised dressings. In emergency, use cleanest cloth available.

Triangular bandage: Very useful. Make from muslin, sheet, clean cloth, about 40 inches square; cut diagonally to make two bandages. *Fold* to make strong, long bandages (cravat bandage) of desired width.

Universal protective dressing: Pending medical aid, serves to cover and protect limb wounds, as splint in fractures, pressure treatment of burns.

Layer of sterile gauze (covering compress if open wound). Then, 1-inch layer absorbent cotton.

Wrap with several layers of muslin or clean cloth.

Cover with waterproof plastic film, such as transparent film used for food wrapping.

Common bandages

Triangular bandage for scalp or forehead

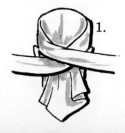
1.

2.

3.

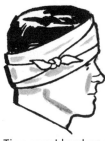

Tie a cravat bandage over a compress covering wound of ear or head.

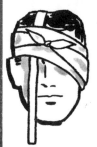 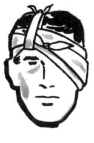

Use cravat bandage to protect an injured eye. Snug but not tight.

For injured palm, wrap cravat around hand, leaving thumb out. ↓

Carry lower end of bandage back of hand, ← around base of thumb.

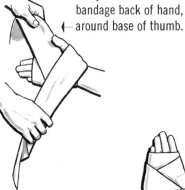

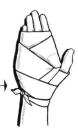

Wrap remaining ends → of bandage around hand and fingers; tie.

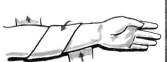

Start spiral bandage on small part of injured limb.

To begin finger bandage, anchor one end of gauze at the wrist.

Wrap spiral bandage as far up injured limb as needed.

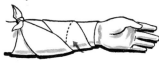

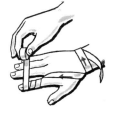

Wrap bandage in spiral down finger, then back to wrist; tie at wrist.

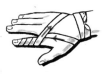

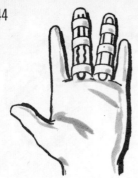

Tape any small splint to broken finger.

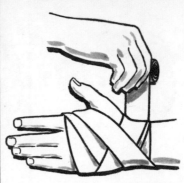

Wrap figure-eight bandage to protect injured hand or wrist.

Use triangular bandage for hand or foot. To stop palm bleeding, clench wad of gauze with fingers, tie bandage on fist.

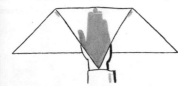 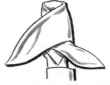

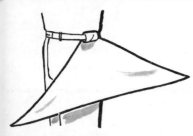

Cover hip or groin injury with large triangular bandage. Tuck top of bandage under a belt, tie bottom ends around leg.

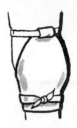

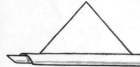

Begin torso bandage by rolling large base of triangle up part way.

Tie rolled part at waist, put point of triangle over shoulder; adjust bandage to cover wound.

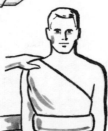

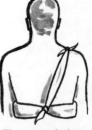

Tie extra cloth to top; tie free end at back of waist.

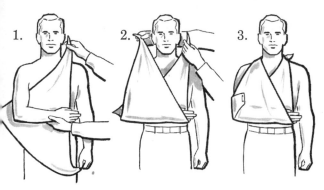

Use triangular bandage to make arm sling. Tie behind neck, but be sure knot isn't directly over spine. Pin corner at elbow. If forearm is injured, elevate hand slightly above level of elbow.

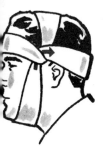

To bandage cheek or ear, start with middle of bandage over compress at wound. Cross ends at opposite side of head, tie over the compress.

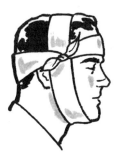

To hold compress on elbow (or knee) use cravat bandage at least 8 inches wide. Bend elbow to right angle. Place middle of bandage over elbow, wrap as shown, and tie.

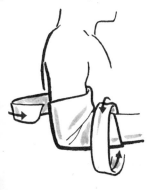
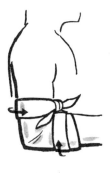

Transporting the injured

Moving broken neck victim

Always use a
flat, rigid
"stretcher"—
Door
Shutter
Board
Ladder

Do not move before medical aid arrives unless essential.

Put rigid "stretcher" such as door alongside victim. One person kneels at head, grasps victim's head firmly between both hands, steadies it so it does not twist in any direction. Helpers grasp victim's clothing at hips and shoulders and *slide* him carefully onto stretcher. *Move his entire body* as if patient were stiff as a log, no bending anywhere.

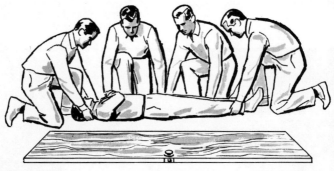

Do not allow
victim's head
and neck to
tilt or twist

If broken neck victim is lying on face, or crumpled: One person kneels and grasps victim's head at jaw angles, exerts traction so head does not turn or move. Then a helper gently straightens and supports legs. One or two other helpers gently turn body onto stretcher—head and neck turning in unison.

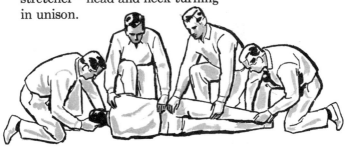

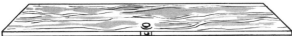

Put rolled cloth, sweater, pads around sides of head to prevent rolling. No pillow under head. Fold victim's arms, tie body to board stretcher.

If not sure whether victim has broken neck or broken back, treat as broken neck.

Grasp sides of head; exert gentle traction on injured neck

Always place broken neck victim face up

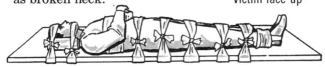

Moving broken back victim

Treat same as for broken neck except that pad to conform to shape of natural curve or "hollow" of back is needed if board stretcher

Board should be at least 15 inches wide and 5 feet long

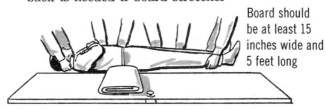

is used. It is relatively easy to put broken back victim *face down* on a blanket, and transport. Keep him face down if transferred to ordinary stretcher.

Vehicle

If *ambulance* is not available and patient *must* be transported some distance, try to get a truck or station wagon with flat floor; pad will ease jolts. If passenger car must be used, remove rear cushion or use board or padding material to make bed on which patient lies full-length. Don't "jackknife" patient into seat unless you are certain his injuries are slight. Jolts, bumps, sudden stops are dangerous; drive cautiously.

Blanket stretcher

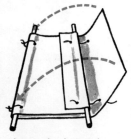

Improvised stretcher

Blanket, rug, canvas, folded over poles. Tie. Test strength

For patients (*except* broken neck or back) who must be lifted or carried in lying down position. If broken bones, *splint* before moving. Blanket with edges rolled (or rug, or other stout fabric) is usually simplest stretcher to improvise, for *carrying* or *lifting* patient.

Tuck folded blanket edge against patient. Turn him slightly away, very carefully push blanket under him as far as possible. Turn him back to center of blanket, pull edge through.

Roll both edges of blanket toward patient in center. Rolled edges give firm grasp for carrying or lifting. Two bearers at each side, preferably three.

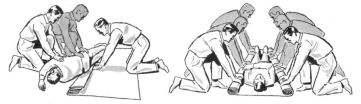

Push edge under victim   Grasp rolled edges; lift

Carrying without a stretcher

When victim need not be carried in lying down position. Consider nature of injury. *Never* use these for broken neck or broken back patient.

Three persons kneel, slide hands under victim's body, lift him to their knees in unison, then rise to their feet while turning victim toward their chests. Work as a unit, co-ordinate movements.

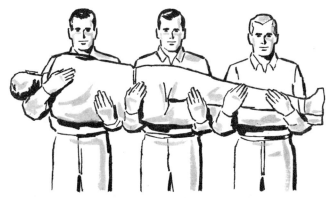

Bearers should keep in step; avoid jarring victim

transporting the injured

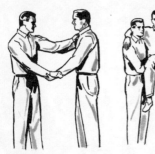 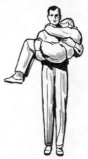

Two persons kneel on sides of victim. Each passes one arm under patient's back, one under his thighs. Bearers grasp each other's wrists and shoulders; rise slowly.

Lift victim by putting one arm under his knees, and other arm firmly around his back. Lean back slightly.

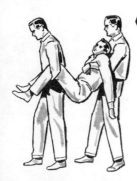

← One bearer clasps his hands around victim's chest. Other bearer puts hands under victim's knees. Bearers lift in unison.

Victim's arms crossed → in front of bearer's shoulders.

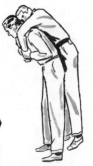

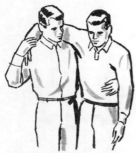 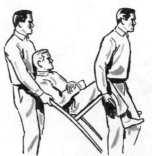

Here's how one bearer can assist a slightly injured person to walk.

Two persons can carry patient on a chair, as shown. Test strength of the chair before lifting.

Wounds, cuts, and bruises

Immediate first aid for major wounds: stop *bleeding*, combat *shock*, keep breathing passages clear of obstruction, and give *artificial respiration* if necessary. Suspect *broken bones*. Keep victim warm and covered. Do not move him unless absolutely necessary (see *Transporting the injured*). Elevate wounded limb unless fractured. Give no stimulants until bleeding stops. Cover wound with sterile dressing or clean cloth and get doctor at once. Do not use antiseptics unless told to by doctor. See specific headings in this book.

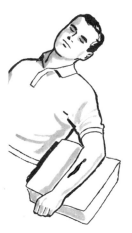

Elevate limb; apply pressure to wound

Abdominal injuries

"*Closed*" *wounds* of abdomen (no break in skin) are easily overlooked. Suspect if victim has suffered severe blow, fall, or crushing injury of abdomen. May be internal bleeding. Little can be done until surgeon explores. Keep patient warm, lying on back. Give nothing by mouth, not even water. Get doctor at once.

Keep victim of abdominal injury flat on back; give no fluids

"*Open*" *wound* of abdomen— deep wound, cut, stab, shot. Sterile dressing or clean cloth

wounds, cuts, and bruises

over wound to draw edges together, stop bleeding, give protection. May be internal bleeding. Get doctor at once. Keep patient lying flat on back, warm. See *puncture wounds*.

Protruding intestines

Important →

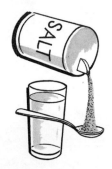

Quickly prepare warm salt water

Exposed intestines *must not be allowed to dry out*. This could be fatal. Cover immediately with large sterile dressing and bandage (or clean cloth in emergency) which *must be kept constantly moist*. Use warm salt water to moisten, preferably, boiled water with 1 teaspoonful of salt to pint. In emergency, use cleanest water you can get; intestines must not dry for an instant. Do not try to put intestines back in place. Give nothing by mouth. Keep patient warm, on back, knees bent with rolled blanket or coat under knees. Get doctor at once.

Abrasions
(*Skinned knee, scraped elbow*)

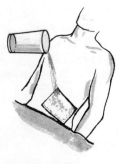

Do not permit delicate exposed parts to dry

Scraped skin surface bleeds or oozes blood. If coarse bits of dirt are in wound, pick out with small tweezers sterilized by passing through match or gas flame. Rub gently with bar of plain mild soap under running water, or wash lavishly with soap and water and clean cloth or pieces of sterile gauze or cotton (fresh piece for each swabbing). Rinse under running tap water. Cover with sterile dressing or adhesive bandage. If dirt is ground into wound, see doctor.

Blisters
Water blisters; blood blisters

Caused by pinching, rubbing, or chafing skin. If blister is small, unbroken, not likely to be injured: wash gently with soap and water, cover with sterile gauze or adhesive compress; leave alone until fluids are absorbed naturally.

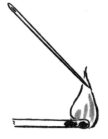

Sterilize needle by holding in a flame

A large blister is likely to be broken or to rupture spontaneously. Anticipate this by opening blister. Sterilize needle by holding in flame. Puncture edge of blister at two points. Press with sterile gauze to force out fluid. Cover with sterile dressing or adhesive bandage. Do *not* open blisters caused by major burns.

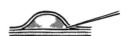

Wash blister; puncture it at the edge

If blistered skin has been rubbed off, exposing raw surface: Clean with warm soap and water and sterile cotton swabs. Cover with sterile dressing. Watch for signs of infection (spreading redness, radiating red lines, pus). At first signs, see doctor.

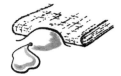

Gently press edge of blister with sterile gauze

Bruises (*Contusions*)

Caused by blows or falls that break small vessels under skin without breaking surface. Injury is first red, then discolored ("black eye" is typical bruise). Minor

wounds, cuts, and bruises

bruises need little first aid. *Caution:* Internal bleeding may accompany bruises of abdomen; other severe bruises may involve broken bones—see doctor. If skin is broken, treat as open wound.

For minor bruises, immediate treatment to relieve pain and limit discoloration is application of cold—ice bags, cloths wrung out of very cold water. *After* a day or so, heat may be applied. Your doctor may think it helpful to try newer enzyme treatments which may reduce swollen discolorations quite rapidly.

Chest wounds
(*"Sucking" injuries*)

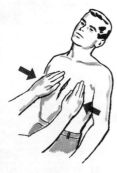

Immediately push together edges of deep chest wound

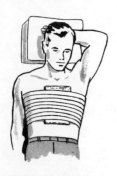

Bind compress over wound; place pad under shoulders

Crushing blows, punctures, stabs, gunshot wounds may create an opening from lungs to outside air. Air may enter and blow out of the wound with "sucking" or hissing sounds. Froth or bubbles may be seen. Stop up this opening *immediately*. Put your hands at each side of wound, push together as victim exhales, to plug the opening. Cover wound with compress and bandage to make airtight, bind firmly. Have victim lie down but keep his shoulders slightly raised, supported with pads, torso turned toward injured side. Get doctor at once.

Give nothing by mouth. Do not attempt to lessen shock by elevating feet, if doing so makes breathing more difficult.

Cuts *and* **scratches**

If small, minor:

Wash well with soap and clean cloth or cotton swabs dipped into warm soapy water.

Rinse under running water from faucet or poured from pitcher (city tap water is safe).

Cover with adhesive bandage or sterile gauze held by adhesive tape.

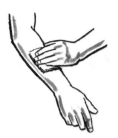

Wash minor cuts with soap; rinse; cover with a sterile bandage

If deep, extensive:

Don't apply medicines.

Control bleeding by hand pressure over gauze pad, clean cloth or handkerchief, until doctor arrives. Tie bandage over sterile dressing if help is delayed.

If skin around wound is grossly dirty, and patient is far from medical help, clean gently with soap and water after bleeding stops, washing *away* from wound. Other dirt such as grease may be removed by naphtha, kerosene (never motor fuel—contains lead) or rubbing alcohol.

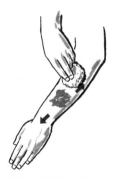

Deep cuts may need stitches to minimize scars—always get medical aid.

Wait until bleeding stops to wash dirt out of deep wounds

Gunshot wounds

Control bleeding, think of fractures; treat like other wounds. Don't probe, or put antiseptics into wound. Also see *puncture wounds.*

wounds, cuts, and bruises

Puncture wounds
Penetrating, perforating injuries

Inflicted by relatively small objects driven under skin, sometimes deeply, or entirely through body, leaving entrance and exit wounds (perforating wounds). Examples: stepping on nail; bullets or shot; wood, glass, or metal splinters; particles driven by firecrackers, firearms or other types of explosions.

A small puncture wound may be washed with soap and water, rinsed under running water. Cover with dressing or adhesive bandage. But the entrance point of a puncture wound is usually small, bleeds little. It cannot be cleaned in depth. It is useless to try to force antiseptics into the wound. Do not attempt it.

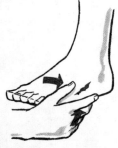

Gently squeeze edges of small puncture, to encourage bleeding

Treat like other wounds according to immediate emergency (shock, fracture). *Encourage* bleeding to "wash out" wound from inside, by gentle pressure around its edges, if you are sure this will not cause further injury.

Important → *Always* see doctor for treatment of puncture wounds. There is danger of tetanus (lockjaw) from organisms which may be carried into the body.

Never remove a projecting object such as a rod or wood splinter that is deeply buried in the body. It may be plugging injured vessels. Removal may cause serious or fatal bleeding.

Splinters

How to remove small splinters, thorns, near surface of skin: Wash with soapy water. Sterilize large needle, knife blade or tweezers by holding in open flame. Press needle against skin near point of splinter. Scrape and dig gently to push splinter out. Loosened splinter may be grasped at end by tweezers and pulled out at same angle it entered flesh. "Milk" surrounding flesh to encourage bleeding. Cover with sterile compress. If imbedded, see doctor.

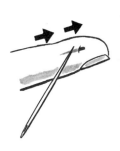

Scrape small splinters out with a sterilized needle

Prevent cuts, scratches, penetrating injuries

Teach children not to run with or throw sharp objects. . . . Don't leave cutlery or sharp-edged tools lying around—keep in separate storage compartments. . . . Keep home workshop power tools disconnected—lock switches, power supply, so children can't turn on. . . . If guns are kept in house, keep them locked up, unloaded. . . . Keep a clean yard, free of bottles, cans, broken glass, boards, nails, wire.

← Keep home safe

Fishhook in flesh

If accident occurs far from aid, and if fishhook is not imbedded in critical area such as face or near eye, remove as follows:

Press down on shank of hook

If doctor is soon available, have him remove fishhook

wounds, cuts, and bruises

until barbed end pushes through the skin and is free (a slight incision at point where tip emerges makes it easier). Cut off barbed end with pliers, clippers. Remove shaft of hook. Wash wound with soap and water, encourage bleeding, cover with dressing or adhesive bandage, see doctor as soon as possible.

If hook is in critical area or has caused much damage, cover wound with sterile dressing, protect with soft bandaging, see doctor as soon as possible. All puncture wounds should be seen by doctor because of danger of tetanus.

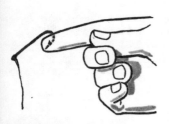

1. Don't pull on hook.

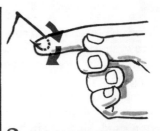

2. Push barb on through.

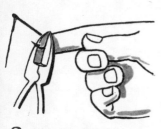

3. Clip off barb.

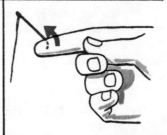

4. Remove shaft of hook.

Sprains, strains, and dislocations

Sprains

A sprain results from tearing ligaments which hold bones together at joints. It may be hard to distinguish between a sprain and a fracture—both may result from same injury. If any doubt, handle as fracture (see *Broken bones*). Symptoms of sprain:

Pain in joint, increases on movement. Tenderness to touch.

Rapid swelling.

Black and blue discoloration (may not appear for several hours).

Immediate aid:

Send for doctor.

Relieve pain by resting joint. Movement may be dangerous.

Elevate sprained joint higher than rest of body, so it gets less blood. Give support—pillow, padded clothing.

Bandage to prevent unnecessary motion if patient has to walk. Loosen the bandage if swelling increases.

For first few hours after injury, apply ice bag or cold compresses. This contracts vessels, minimizes

Supports for
Sprained Joints:

ELBOW, WRIST
Arm in sling

KNEE, ANKLE
Padding under leg to elevate about a foot higher than body

Caution: Back "sprain" may be fracture

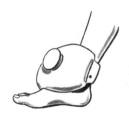

Ice bag may
help relieve pain
and swelling

sprains, strains, and dislocations

swelling, eases pain. *After* a day or so, if doctor is not available, change to *hot* compresses. Do not apply heat immediately after the injury.

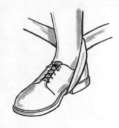

Place middle of bandage under shoe in front of heel

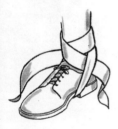

Cross ends at back of heel and in front, over instep

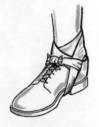

Loop each end under rear of bandage; tie over instep

Sprained ankle

If injury occurs far from help or it is absolutely essential for a sprained ankle to bear weight, a snug ankle bandage gives support for walking. *Never* walk with a sprained ankle (might be broken) unless in serious emergency.

Leave shoe on, loosen laces. Place long bandage under shoe in front of heel. Bring bandage ends behind and above heel, cross, bring forward and cross over instep. Tuck ends under loops formed by first step of bandaging, on each side of foot. Pull ends together, tie over instep.

Strains

A strain is caused by overstretching or "pulling" muscles or tendons. Back strain ("crick in the back") is common. Symptoms:

Sharp pain or "stitch" at time of injury.

Stiffness and soreness get worse in a few hours.

Pain on movement.

How to help:

Put injured part at rest. Sit or lie in most comfortable position.

Apply heat in any form—hot water bottle, lamp, heating pad.

Give gentle massage with warm rubbing alcohol or witch hazel. Rub toward the heart.

If pain eases sufficiently, rub more forcefully, knead gently, to help loosen stiffened muscles.

See doctor if back strain is severe. May need strapping.

Prevent back strain

Low back strain is most often caused by improper lifting technique, or attempting to lift objects that are too heavy. The most important lifting rule is never to let the lower back arch forward. Do not bend over stiff-legged to lift object from floor—place your feet close to object, crouch with back straight, feet flat on floor; grasp object firmly; lift slowly using thigh muscles.

Don't lean over projection such as radiator to lift stuck window. Don't reach to pick up something when one arm is loaded with baby or packages. Get help if object to be lifted is heavy. Don't push or lift if footing is insecure—a slip or twist may wrench your back.

Sudden, quick lifting of heavy objects is dangerous, especially if you are unaccustomed to it. Do not keep on trying to lift an object if you feel a slight discomfort in your back. Take frequent rests if repeated heavy lifts must be made.

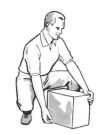

Bend legs to lift

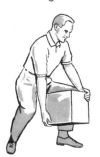

Keep back flat

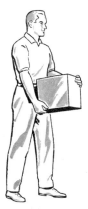

Lift slowly

62

Dislocations

A blow, fall, sudden twisting may force a bone out of place at a joint, causing a *dislocation*. Indications:

Joint looks out of shape compared to similar joint.

Swelling, usually rapid.

Pain and tenderness at site.

Patient can't move joint or motion is limited.

May be *shock*.

Immediate First Aid:

Send for doctor.

Do not try to straighten out joint or force bone back in place (except jaw, finger, toe dislocations; see below).

Suspect that bones *may* be fractured. In general, handle as if part were fractured (see *Broken bones*).

Put patient in comfortable position. Keep weight off injured part. Give gentle support to injured part.

Apply ice bag or cloths wrung out of very cold water, to ease pain and minimize swelling.

Finger or toe dislocation

Grasp with one hand on each side of dislocated joint. Slowly pull free end of finger or toe in a straight line until it snaps in place. Do not use great force. If one or two attempts fail, wait for doctor. Do

Support for
Dislocations:

ELBOW, SHOULDER, WRIST
Arm in sling (not pulled up tightly)

ANKLE
Often accompanied by fracture. Pillow splint

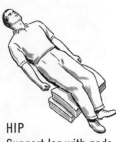

HIP
Support leg with pads in position in which patient holds it. Transport as for broken back

KNEE
Padding under knee in position in which patient holds it

not try to reduce large joint at base of thumb or great toe joint. Don't pull dislocated finger or toe if an open wound is near the dislocated joint. Dress the wound and get medical aid.

Jaw dislocation

In an emergency a first-aider may try to correct a dislocated jaw. Symptoms: Lower jaw sags down, patient cannot close mouth.

Wrap your thumbs with cloth to protect them. Face patient, put your thumbs in his mouth on lower back teeth, your fingers under his chin. Press firmly down and back with your thumbs, upward with your fingers under his chin. Get your thumbs out fast to prevent injury when jaw snaps back in place.

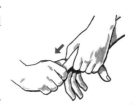

Do not pull hard while trying to put finger back in place

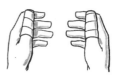

Wrap thumbs with cloth before pushing on dislocated jaw

Seat patient in chair; stand directly in front

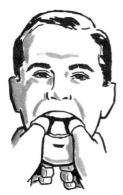

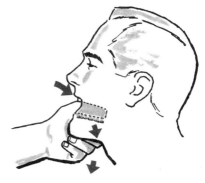

Place thumbs on lower rear teeth; fingers under chin

Press down and back with thumbs, pull up with fingers under chin. Don't let jaw snap shut on thumbs.

Burns

Minor burns

Hold immediately under cold running water for several minutes. Or, immerse in container of clean cool water.

Cleanse with plain white soap and water.

For mild burns of moderate size: Apply a paste of wet baking soda. Or gauze, impregnated with petroleum jelly, sold in sterile packets. Or a mild burn ointment. Ointments should be used *only* on minor burns.

Cover with sterile bandage.

Immediate exclusion of air gives greatest pain relief of burns.

Major burns

Immediate step whenever possible: Wrap patient carefully in blanket or sheet and get to hospital at once.

If first step is not possible:

Immerse burned part (leg, arm) in *warm*, not hot, water. If burn is extensive or involves trunk, thighs, large skin areas, put patient (clothes and all) into bathtub full of warm running water.

This excludes air from burn and helps prevent shock. Stir some baking soda into the water.

Remove clothing carefully. Use scissors to *cut around cloth* that

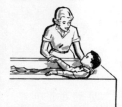

Warm running water

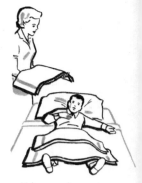

sticks to burned skin. *Never* pull clothing that adheres to skin. Leave it. Leave all foreign particles except large ones that come off easily. Keep patient supported in tub until the doctor comes.

If immersion of burned part is not possible, or patient has to be removed from tub, have him lie on bed on freshly laundered sheet. Cover with dry dressings made as thick as possible.

Wrap patient in fresh clean sheet, and cover with blanket to keep him *comfortably* warm while waiting for doctor.

If immersion not possible, put victim on clean sheet; cover. Raise foot of bed 10 inches to lessen shock

Important don'ts

Do not open large blisters.

Do not apply antiseptics.

Do not apply greases, ointments, butter, dressings that are not sterile, fluffy cotton, or any materials the doctor will find hard to remove.

Combat shock

Immediate fluid replacement helps to prevent *shock*, a major threat of severe burns.

Thirst is a sign of impending shock. Give fluids unless patient is unconscious or vomiting. Give this saline *shock solution*:

    1 teaspoon salt

    ½ teaspoon baking soda
       dissolved in

    1 quart water

Do not give fluids too rapidly

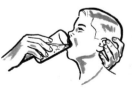

Give fluids if victim is conscious and not vomiting

burns

(may produce vomiting). Give about one cupful every hour.

Bandaging

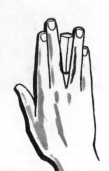

Place clean cloth between badly burned fingers or toes

Bad burns are susceptible to *infection*. Immediate first-aid purpose of bandaging is to hold the dressings in place, exclude air, protect against dirt, germs. Leave more elaborate bandaging to doctor. Prevent raw, burned skin surfaces—between fingers, toes, or under arms—from sticking together by separating surfaces with moistened strips of clean cloth. Cover with sterile bandage until doctor can take over.

Extensive burns

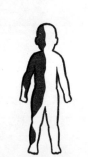

Any burns covering a large area of skin are very serious

Whether superficial or deep, burns which cover any large area such as chest, back, or a complete upper extremity are always major burns. So are burns of face and hands (other than the most trivial) which may leave scars or deformities. Medically, burns that cover any nine per cent of the body surface are extensive. Give immediate first aid; get prompt medical help.

Chemical burns

of body from strong acids, alkalis, corrosive fluids

Strip clothing and drench burn continuously with lavish amounts of clean water. If possible, rush immediately under bathroom shower, turn on forcefully, strip clothing under running shower. If there is delay, corrosive liquid has dried, do not irrigate; summon doctor.

Powder burns
Fireworks, cap pistols

Unless skin is lacerated, torn (see *Wounds, cuts, and bruises*), cleanse gently with bland white soap, water. Cover with dry dressing.

Greatest danger from most powder burns is not the burn itself but tiny puncture wounds of powder particles which may drive *tetanus* organisms deeply into the skin. All children and adults should have tetanus toxoid inoculations which give protection against the disease.

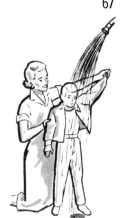

Quickly drench chemical burn with large amounts of water

← Important

Prevent burn tragedies

Keep handles of pots, frying pans turned in on kitchen range. Don't put hot tea, coffee, liquids on a tablecloth or scarf hanging over side of a table—child may pull or run into cloth and tip over steaming liquids. Never leave small child alone in bathtub; he may turn *hot water faucet* and get a bad scald. Place child in tub facing faucet so he won't back into hot metal. Keep tubs, pails, pans of hot water off floor where children may run or trip.

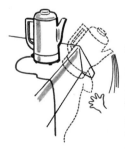

Child may pull tablecloth and upset scalding liquids

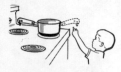

Keep handles of hot
pans out of reach

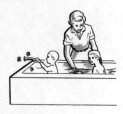

Never leave small
child alone in tub

Don't hold child in your lap while you drink or pass hot beverages. Cover hot pipes, radiators. Keep matches, cigarette lighters out of reach until child is old enough to be taught safe use and dangers. Never leave children alone around a bonfire, outdoor grill, fireplace, glowing coals or open flame. Remember that Christmas trees dry out in the house and are highly inflammable. Never throw water on a grease or oven fire—smother it with salt or soda.

Poisons

Swallowed poisons

Call doctor at once, or prepare to rush patient to nearest hospital if no doctor is available, but first give *immediate* first aid. Don't lose time seeking specific poison antidote. Use simple measures immediately available.

Call doctor, or local Poison Control Center; telephone number_____

If patient is conscious:

First, *before* telephoning doctor, *dilute* the poison by giving large amounts of fluids. The fluids may cause vomiting, which should be encouraged. May be more effective than waiting for the doctor's more efficient stomach pump.

Give fluids to dilute poison

Important
Head lowered for drainage

If patient vomits, put in prone position, head turned and lowered over bed edge, to prevent inhaling vomited material. If a child, hold face downward on your lap, head hanging over. Induce vomiting by tickling back of throat or putting your finger in throat.

Do not induce vomiting if patient has swallowed *lye* or corrosive acids or alkalis (may be burns around face or mouth); or *kerosene, gasoline, or turpentine.*

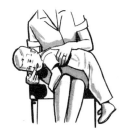

Place child across lap with head down; tickle back of throat

poisons

Emetics
to induce vomiting

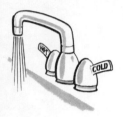

Warm fluids help
to induce vomiting

If patient does not vomit, proceed to *dilute* the poison and *wash out* the stomach by giving *large amounts of fluids* which have emetic (vomiting-inducing) ef- fects. *Speed* is important and it is better to give patient *warm milk or water* than to lose time hunting for materials to mix a more potent emetic. It is easier to induce vom- iting when stomach is full. Try again after giving fluids.

Give glass of milk immediately

Give several glasses of emetic fluids such as:
Warm tap water
Warm salt water (1 teaspoon salt to glass)
Warm mustard water (1 tea- spoon dry mustard to glass)

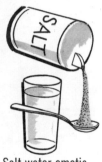

Salt water emetic

Keep giving fluids until vomited liquid is as clear as when swal- lowed. *Do not* force liquids on a semiconscious patient.
After the stomach is emptied, a large dose of *Epsom salts* is good for almost any poison.

Do not rely on antidotes alone

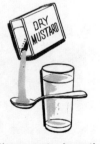

Warm mustard emetic

Always call the doctor. Then give antidote which helps to counter- act the poison. If you do not know what the patient has swallowed, a "universal antidote" is a useful emergency measure.

A *universal antidote* for unknown poisons can be bought at drugstores, kept on hand for emergencies. It consists of:

Pulverized charcoal (activated charcoal)—2 tablespoons
Tannic acid—1 tablespoon
Magnesium oxide—1 tablespoon

Mix in ½ glass of water; give to patient.

Keep universal antidote on hand for emergencies

General antidotes

A similar "homemade" *universal antidote* can be made as follows:

Finely crushed burnt toast—2 tablespoons
Very strong tea—1 tablespoon
Milk of magnesia—1 tablespoon

Mix in ½ glass of water; give to patient.

Make antidote from burnt toast, tea, milk of magnesia

The label of the bottle or package from which the poison has come may list a *specific antidote*. Give this *if immediately available* but do not waste time—it is always safe to give a *universal antidote* first.

Antidote for unknown poisons

Other *quick household antidotes* which help to dilute, absorb, and counteract many kinds of poisons include:

A glass of milk
Two or three raw egg whites beaten into a glass of water
Starch or flour made into a thin "soup" with water

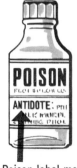

Poison label may list antidote

poisons

(*Do not* give milk, oily or fatty substances in cases of suspected *phosphorus* poisoning.)

Save the bottle, box, or container from which the patient obtained the poison. Save unconsumed portion of the suspected liquid, tablet, powder, or particle. Save labels giving brand names and name of manufacturer. If a drug overdose, save *prescription number and name of pharmacist*. Show to doctor or take with you to hospital so the *poison can be identified* and emergency medical treatment beyond the range of simple first aid can be begun.

Give poison container to → doctor or hospital

Keep warm, keep breathing

If the suspected poisoning victim is unconscious, semicomatose, shows signs of shock or difficulty in breathing:

Keep air passages open. Keep patient in prone (on stomach) position with head low, turned to one side. Wipe mucous secretions from mouth with handkerchief or finger. Keep tongue from falling back and blocking air passage. Lift nape of neck, put your hand under jaw, pull jaw forward and upward to extend neck and tilt head backward.

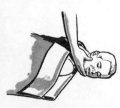

Place victim on stomach, head turned to side

Watch for slowed or stopped breathing. If breathing stops, give immediate *mouth to mouth resuscitation* (see page 10).

Keep patient warm, covered. Do not give stimulants.

Quick-use chart
of common poison antidotes

Some poisoning symptoms are immediate, dramatic, and acute; others may be rather long-delayed. Homes, plants, and offices contain hundreds of necessary and indispensable materials which may be mildly or seriously toxic if swallowed. Young children put things into their mouths while exploring the world and are particularly liable to poisoning from large overdoses of simple household remedies and prescription drugs, which are beneficial and harmless when properly used. Always call doctor if poisoning is suspected. Do not wait for symptoms to appear. Give *immediate* first aid. Give fluids. It is safe to give a dose of *universal antidote* immediately, and a *quick glass of milk* almost always does much good.

Always get medical aid if poisoning suspected; quickly give antidote or milk

Combined ingredients of *universal antidote* act against common poisons in the same general way as more concentrated and specific antidotes. *If the cause of the poisoning is known*, and immediate first aid has been given, more specific steps may be taken while *medical aid is on the way*.

The following chart gives additional first-aid instructions and lists helpful antidotes for some common causes of poisoning. Continue these steps until medical aid is available.

Alkalis,
caustic

Lye
Ammonia
Drainpipe cleaners
Quicklime
Washing soda

Do not force vomiting
Give acid fruit juices, such as juice of 4 lemons in pint of water
Or, slightly diluted vinegar
Follow with two or three raw egg whites in water
Or, salad oil, cooking oil, melted butter
Or, glass or two of milk

Acids,
strong

Battery acid
Sulfuric
Nitric
Hydrochloric

Do not force vomiting
Teacupful of milk of magnesia
Or, 2 tablespoons of baking soda in pint of water
Then, raw egg whites in water
Or, glass or two of milk
Or, salad oil, any vegetable oil, about ¼ glass

Carbolic acid

Phenol
(Ingredient
of common
disinfectants)
Creosote
Creosol disinfectants

Give soapsuds immediately
Or, give Epsom salts (2 tablespoons to pint of water)
Then, large amounts luke-warm water (*Do not* give any strong emetic)
Also, give thin "soup" of flour or cornstarch in water
Or, raw egg whites in water
Do not give alcoholic drinks

Iodine

Flour or cornstarch in water; bread; large amounts of starchy substances
Follow with emetic; induce vomiting
Repeat starch and emetic until returned material has no blue color

Petroleum distillates

Kerosene
Gasoline
Benzine
Naphtha
Lighter fluid
Inflammable
cleaning fluids

Do not force vomiting (danger of aspiration pneumonia)
Give half-cup of mineral oil
Stimulant; strong coffee, tea
Keep warm, combat shock
Artificial respiration if necessary

Salicylate drug overdose

Aspirin
Headache and
cold pills
Oil of wintergreen

Induce vomiting unless it has occurred
Give *universal antidote*
Or, *weak* baking soda solution (1 teaspoon to pint)
Strong coffee

"Sleep drug" overdose

Barbiturates
Sedatives
Opiates
Codeine
Morphine
Paregoric

If conscious, give emetic, induce vomiting
Strong black coffee
Keep patient awake—slap face with wet towel, walk him about, but do not exhaust him
Artificial respiration if necessary

Wood alcohol

Rubbing alcohol
Denatured alcohol
Methanol

Emetic; induce vomiting
Give tablespoon of baking soda in quart of warm water
Repeat emetic, soda solution
Follow with glass of milk containing teaspoon of baking soda

Prevent poisoning tragedies

Be aware that many essential household articles are potentially toxic if accidentally swallowed or misused: disinfectants, lye, ammonia, flammable and noninflammable cleaning fluids, insecticides, bleaches, rat poisons, moth balls, kerosene, gasoline, turpentine, paint thinners, household remedies and prescription drugs in overdosage. If there are small children in the house, keep such articles *on a high shelf* well out of reach, or preferably in a *locked cabinet. Never* put such things into a soft drink bottle, cup, or any container associated with food—a sip can be swallowed before it can be spit out. Never put anything on food shelves except food. Keep drugs and home remedies, even "harmless" ones, locked up. Do not leave pills in a *handbag* or low *drawer;* children love to rummage. Never tell a child that a pill is candy or "tastes like candy." Never take a medicine until you have *read the label*. If label is gone or illegible, discard bottle.

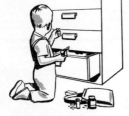

Never leave pills or medicines in low drawer or handbag

Food poisoning

Do not assume that all severe intestinal upsets which occur after eating are due to food poisoning. Appendicitis, other illnesses may cause similar symptoms. *Suspect* food poisoning if more than one person becomes ill after eating

Symptoms of food poisoning may be similar to those of other illnesses

the same foods which were improperly prepared or spoiled.

The most common forms of food poisoning are infections caused by *bacteria* or their toxins in contaminated foods. Symptoms may be very mild, last only a few hours, or very severe with urgent need of medical aid. Most bacterial food poisonings are caused by *staphylococci* (germ family that causes boils and abscesses) or *salmonella* organisms.

Staphylococcal food poisoning may cause symptoms almost immediately, commonly within 2 to ← Illness may not begin until a day 4 hours after eating. Symptoms of or two after eating *salmonella* poisoning usually are contaminated food longer delayed—from 6 hours after eating to a day or even two days later. Recovery commonly takes longer; chills, fever; can be serious; get doctor.

If these symptoms occur, call doctor:

Abdominal pain and distress
Abdomen is always *soft*, never rigid or board-like
Nausea and vomiting
Cramps
Diarrhea
Chills or fever, prostration (salmonella poisoning)

Important Don'ts

Do not give laxatives, cathartics, or *anything* by mouth as long as nausea and vomiting persist.

poisons

After nausea stops
give victim large →
quantities of fluids

First aid:

Put patient to bed, keep warm.

After nausea and vomiting subside, give large quantities of lukewarm water, fluids.

If no diarrhea, salt-water enemas (1 teaspoon of salt to quart of water) may be given.

Botulinus poisoning

Caused by powerful toxins of organisms which may be in *improperly home-canned foods*, especially low-acid foods. Commercially canned foods and home-canned foods canned by the pressure method are safe. Boiling of home-canned foods for 15 minutes before eating insures safety.

Properly canned
foods are safe from
botulinus toxins

Recognize symptoms and call doctor at once

These symptoms commonly begin 18 to 24 hours after eating the food but *may* not appear for several days:

Great fatigue

May be no nausea or vomiting

Predominant nervous system symptoms:

Dizziness

Headache

Disturbances of vision, blurring, double vision

Difficulty in breathing, swallowing, and speaking

Muscular weakness

Temperature may be subnormal

Mushroom poisoning

Put patient to bed in quiet room; *very serious!*

    Call doctor immediately.

    No test can prove unknown mushrooms to be safe and edible. Avoid *all* wild mushrooms.

    The following symptoms of mushroom poisoning may appear within a few minutes to 2 or 3 hours after eating, or within 8 to 15 hours, depending upon the variety of fungus:

Abdominal pain
Diarrhea
Dizziness
Derangement of vision
Cold sweating
Cramps in arms or legs

← Emergency

First Aid:

Give large dose of Epsom salts. *Call doctor* at once or take patient to hospital.

Weed and plant poisoning

Leaves, roots, berries, seeds and other parts of many weeds, wild plants, and garden plants (foxglove, monkshood, rhubarb *leaves*, lilies, others) may be toxic if eaten. *Teach* children not to eat strange berries, fruits or plant parts; avoid them yourself. *Symptoms* of plant poisoning vary; usually include abdominal pain, cramps, nausea, vomiting (may be juice stains around mouth).

← Caution children not to eat unfamiliar wild berries, fruits

poisons   # Immediate treatment

Induce vomiting immediately if it has not occurred.

Give large amounts of fluids, milk if available.

Give dose of Epsom salts.

Give *universal antidote*.

Save specimen of plant or part thought to have caused poisoning; show to doctor.

Prevent food poisoning

Insanitary food handling, lack of refrigeration, keeping foods at room temperature or warmer for several hours, underlie most cases of food poisoning. Food handlers

Proper food handling and refrigeration help to prevent food poisoning

→ with cut fingers, colds, and boils may introduce germs which can multiply rapidly in *foods that are not thoroughly cooked or are heated very little*, such as salads, meringues, salad dressings, creamed dishes, custard fillings, cold cuts. *Refrigeration* retards growth of germs. If no refrigeration available, consume foods *soon after preparation;* discard *leftovers* that have stood exposed to room or outdoor air and warmth for hours. On *picnics, car trips, camping trips*, keep food in portable icebox. On *vacations*, only raw (unpasteurized) milk may be obtainable. You can *pasteurize milk* by bringing it to a rolling boil, plunging pan into ice cubes for rapid cooling (has slightly "cooked" flavor). A better way, if you have a thermometer and double boiler, is as follows:

Bring water to boil in bottom half of double boiler.

Put milk in top half of boiler (over boiling water), insert thermometer into milk, stir milk until thermometer registers 160 degrees. Hold at that temperature for 15 seconds.

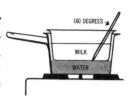

Keep milk at 160 degrees for 15 seconds

Cool milk *rapidly* by placing container in ice cubes, or changes of cold water. Keep stirring until temperature drops to 50 degrees.

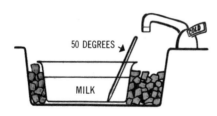

Cool milk quickly in ice or cold water; stir until temperature drops to 50 degrees

Bites
and
stings

VENOMOUS BITE

Puncture marks

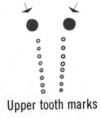

Upper tooth marks

Lower tooth marks

NONVENOMOUS

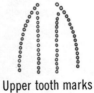

Upper tooth marks

Lower tooth marks

Snake bite

Venomous and nonvenomous

Venomous snakes of the United States are pit vipers (rattlers, copperheads, moccasins), except for the rare coral snake of Southern regions.

The "bite" of a venomous snake usually leaves *two* small puncture marks, as shown.

There may be *one* puncture mark if the snake struck at an angle, or sometimes three or four puncture marks. The "bite" is really a hypodermic injection through hollow fangs which deposit venom. Smaller teeth behind the fangs may cause rows of scratches in addition to the larger puncture marks.

Swelling may obscure the puncture marks. Pain at the site of most venomous bites is immediate and intense.

Nonpoisonous snake bite usually leaves two U-shaped rows of fine tooth marks, as shown. There is little pain or swelling.

The bite of a coral snake closely resembles those of nonvenomous snakes. A coral snake bite usually is accompanied by very little pain.

For *nonpoisonous* snake bite, cleanse with plain soap and water, cover with sterile dressing; see doctor.

Poisonous snake bite

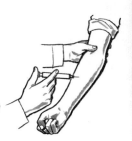

Give antivenin injection if doctor not soon available

The only specific measure for venomous snake bite is injection of antivenin as soon as possible to neutralize the venom. "Snake-bite kits" containing antivenin, instruments, instructions, can be bought at drugstores, sometimes rented on returnable basis by campers and outdoorsmen from pharmacies in "snake country." First aiders can give antivenin injections—*the sooner the better*—although it is best to have a doctor do it unless time would be lost.

If antivenin is not on hand: Immobilize the victim. Have him lie down, keep quiet, no walking or muscular action that can be avoided. *Do not give whiskey or* ← Keep victim quiet, *stimulants*. Ice water, cold cloths, lying down; give no may ease pain but do not stop stimulants or whiskey spread of venom. *Carry* the victim —on stretcher if possible, or on one's back with bitten part hanging down—to nearest doctor or source of help where physician with antivenin can be summoned *urgently*. If there is no possibility of getting medical aid, use the incision-suction method.

bites and stings

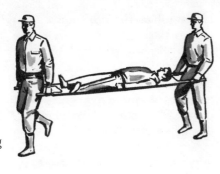

When snake bite victim must be moved, keep him lying down if possible.

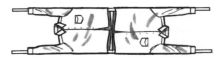

Make an emergency stretcher from two shirts, two poles.

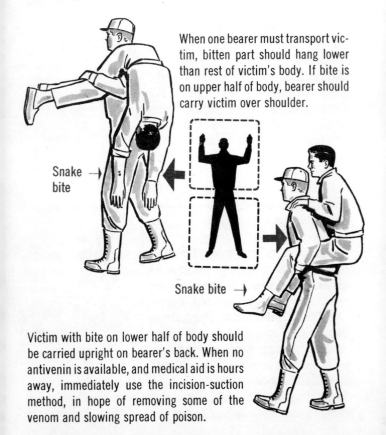

When one bearer must transport victim, bitten part should hang lower than rest of victim's body. If bite is on upper half of body, bearer should carry victim over shoulder.

Snake bite →

Snake bite →

Victim with bite on lower half of body should be carried upright on bearer's back. When no antivenin is available, and medical aid is hours away, immediately use the incision-suction method, in hope of removing some of the venom and slowing spread of poison.

Incision-suction method

For centuries the only recognized (or available) method of treating venomous snake bite was by incision, suction, and tourniquet, thought to remove venom or slow its absorption. Many physicians use this first-aid method, and the armed forces recommend it.

The standard incision-suction technique consists of: A constricting band (loosened every quarter-hour) between wound and body; cuts to induce bleeding at site of ← bite and swollen edges; suction through these cuts by mouth or suction cup.

Use a sharp, sterile knife; make short, shallow cuts directly over puncture marks

Do not apply tourniquet tightly. Its purpose is to slow blood flow, not stop it.

Make the cuts no deeper than ⅜-inch, and even more shallow on hands to avoid cutting nerves. Apply a pressure bandage if an artery is cut accidentally.

Insect bites
Pain and itch relief

Apply ice or wet dressings; hold under cold water. Make a paste of baking soda moistened with water, cover burn or sting site. Apply diluted household ammonia to bite and surrounding skin. Calamine lotion and rubbing alcohol or lotions containing alcohol help to relieve itching. Do not scratch an insect bite. Scratching may result in infection.

bites and stings

Tick bites
Don't touch with bare fingers!

Some ticks spread diseases such as Rocky Mountain spotted fever, tularemia, and relapsing fever. A tick often can be felt before it starts to burrow under the skin, but after it begins to suck it usually cannot be felt. Examine skin and clothing after a day in tick-infested country.

The head of a tick tenaciously resists removal from skin. Don't try to remove ticks with unprotected fingers or allow crushed parts or juices to contact the skin. It may help to make ticks "let go" if you:

Save tick; show it to doctor or local health authorities

Coat them with nail polish, petroleum jelly, or grease. Smother them with kerosene, turpentine, or gasoline. Remove them carefully with tweezers.

Afterward, wash site thoroughly with soap and water.

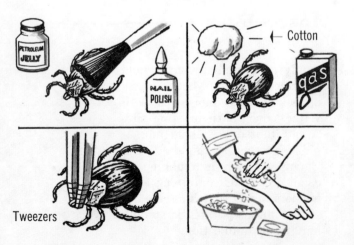

Cotton

Tweezers

Stings:

*Bee, wasp, hornet, yellow jacket
Get the stinger out!*

Cold packs containing baking soda are a good home remedy for relief of local discomfort from stings of bees and related insects. Ice cubes, ice bags, give most comfort.

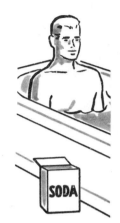

Take lukewarm soda bath if stings are numerous

If you upset a nest of insects, and suffer a "massive dose" of many separate stings, get into a tepid tub bath with a package or more of baking soda stirred into it.

Bees often leave their "stinger" in the center of the sting. The stinging apparatus can be seen as a tiny dark object. It continues to pump venom into the wound after the bee is gone. *Remove the stinger* with an outward scraping motion of a fingernail. *Do not* pinch the stinger between two fingernails or grasp with tweezers. That forces more venom out.

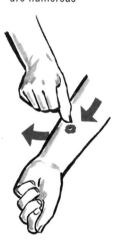

Use fingernail to scrape stinger out of the skin

A few people become so extremely sensitized to insect venom that a sting may cause a serious, even fatal, allergy-like reaction. They should seek medical aid, such as desensitization procedures and emergency steps to take if stung.

Spider bite

Spiders produce venom, but the only common American spider that inflicts a serious bite is the

Beware the red hourglass

bites and stings

Black widow is about ½-inch long with red spot on abdomen

Bite feels like needle prick, and leaves two tiny red marks

black widow. It's a coal-black insect with a pea-size abdomen marked with a reddish hourglass design on its underside.

Its bite causes intense pain, muscle spasm, weak pulse. The pain moves gradually from wound and concentrates in the abdomen.

If these symptoms occur, immediately examine skin for two tiny puncture marks caused by a black widow bite. Call doctor immediately. Save spider for identification, if possible.

Meantime, wash wound with soapsuds, apply baking soda compress, give black coffee as a stimulant, watch for signs of shock (see *Shock*).

Dog bites, cat bites
Other animal bites

Immediate first-aid treatment of animal bites is the same as for other common wounds, except for possibility of rabies (see *rabies*, page 89). Bite injuries range from barely perceptible tooth marks to severe injuries to be treated as major wounds.

Most bites inflicted by dogs, cats, squirrels, rats, mice, and small animals are local soft tissue injuries and immediate first aid aims to prevent infection and promote healing:

1. Cleanse wound thoroughly with soap and water. Preferably, wash under running water with liberal soaping. Paint with antiseptic.

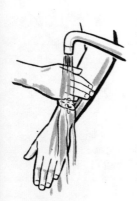

Wash animal bite thoroughly to remove saliva

2. Cover the bite wound with a sterile dressing and bandage.

3. See doctor. *Always* see doctor if bite, no matter how trivial, is on face, head, or neck areas.

Human bites

A human bite may be a real bite or it may be inflicted by teeth that stop the blow of a fist. The human mouth commonly contains varied and virulent bacteria, and serious undermining, spreading infections often follow human bite wounds.

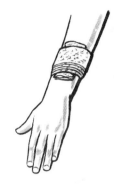

Give first aid, as for animal bites, then have a doctor take over.

Cover bite with sterile dressing; always see doctor

Rabies or hydrophobia

Rabies is a fatal disease which may be transmitted by the saliva of "mad dogs" and infected animals such as cats, squirrels, skunks, foxes, bats, and others.

Most bites are inflicted by healthy animals. An animal that snaps at anything, attacks without provocation, behaves peculiarly or "acts sick," may have rabies.

If bitten, do not become panic-stricken nor fail to take sensible precautions. Give first aid; *have doctor inspect wound;* follow his advice.

Fatality from ← rabies usually can be prevented

Rabies can be prevented by Pasteur treatments (a series of a dozen or more injections) begun after the bite is suffered. Such

**bites
and stings**

treatment can be avoided if the biting animal is kept under observation for a couple of weeks and if it is perfectly healthy at the end of that time. If the animal has been killed, or dies, laboratory examination of its head can usually determine whether it was "mad."

The slow incubation period of rabies usually affords enough time for observation or laboratory tests so that Pasteur treatments need not be started unless tests are positive. Treatments may be started immediately in case of bites of head, neck, shoulders, and hands, but are stopped if the animal proves not to be rabid. If nothing is known about the biting animal, Pasteur treatments may have to be given (depending upon circumstances of the bite) as insurance against a disease which, once established, is invariably fatal. These treatments are almost always effective, if started in time.

Rabies treatment → may have to begin immediately

The doctor's decision depends in part on information you give him and steps you take at the time of the accident.

What to do
if an animal bites you

Important → Capture and confine the biting animal if possible.

Identify the animal and its owner if it belongs in the neighborhood. If a stray, get accurate description so police or dog catcher can track it down.

Do not kill the animal unless absolutely necessary. Do not shoot through head as this may make laboratory studies difficult.

If animal dies or is killed, preserve its head. Your doctor or local health department will tell you what steps to take. Report animal bites to police or authorities according to local regulations.

Prevent many bites and stings

Teach children not to maul or torment pets or tease stray animals. Many nips are inflicted in justifiable self-defense.

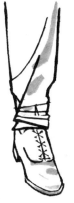

Tie ends of trousers and sleeves to keep out ticks

Wear calf-high boots in snake country; watch your step in woods; probe underbrush with a stick before trampling on it (75 per cent of snake bites occur near the ankle, most of the rest in wrist or hand areas).

Tie shut the open ends of sleeves and trouser legs when strolling through tick-infested grasses and weeds. *Bees and stinging insects* are attracted to dark-colored clothing, tweeds, flannels, sweaty clothing, hair oils and perfumes. If "attacked" by a hostile bee, *move slowly*, don't make jerky movements, slap, or run, unless a whole hive is after you.

Wear gloves when cleaning out a garage to protect against possible black widow bite.

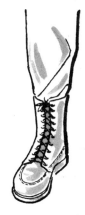

High leather boots give protection against snake bite

Eyes

Chemical burns of eye

Read this now and be ready for *instant action* if dangerous chemicals are splashed or spilled into the eyes. Acids, alkalis, damaging powders and liquids, can cause serious chemical burns of the eye, impaired vision, blindness. Chemicals continue to burn as long as they remain in the eye.

SECONDS COUNT! →
Flush chemicals
from eyes
with water

Immediate flushing out of the chemical minimizes eye damage and may prevent it entirely. Don't waste time trying to find out whether the chemical is an acid or an alkali. It makes no first-aid difference. There's only one thing to remember when dangerous chemicals get into the eyes: *wash out the eyes immediately with large amounts of cool water*.

Hold head under faucet with eye in running stream of cool water. Stream should have good flushing force but not high pressure. Turn head so stream flows over affected eye *away from* unaffected eye. If both eyes are contaminated with chemicals, direct water on both eyes simultaneously or in quick alternation. Flush the eyes thoroughly *before* you take time to call a doctor.

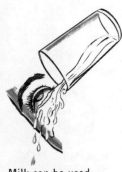

Milk can be used
to wash out eyes
in an emergency

You can't use too much water.

Keep on irrigating the eyes with water for 5 or 10 minutes or until you are very sure that all dangerous chemical material has been washed out. *Remember*, powder particles may be trapped under eyelids. Separate lids gently so water can reach all parts.

DANGER! from lime, cement, lye, battery acids, caustic cleansers that get into eyes

If there's no faucet handy, seize any source of water or any bland fluid you can lay hands on quickly —a bottle of milk will serve in an emergency. Put patient on floor, flat on his back, pour water from pitcher, tumbler, any container, into corner of eye (next to nose) so fluid streams over eyeball and under eyelids. Repeat, repeat, repeat!

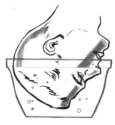

Blink eyes under water to wash out chemicals

Or, eye may be held in stream of water bubbling from drinking fountain. Or, eyes may be submerged in bowl of water while patient keeps blinking them.

Massive, thorough, continuous irrigation! Instant first aid may prevent blindness!

After all chemical materials are washed from eyes, call a doctor. What you do in the *first few seconds* and the next few minutes to wash acids or alkalis from eyes is more important than anything the doctor can do later. After thorough irrigation, put a few drops of clean oil into the eye (mineral oil, castor oil, vegetable oil). This helps to prevent eyelids from sticking to eyeball. Cover both eyes with sterile gauze compress and rush to doctor.

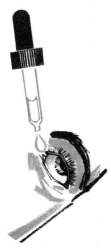

After washing eyes put in a few drops of mineral oil

eyes ## Contusions of eyeball

Hard blows which do not cut or penetrate the eye may "bruise" it internally and can be serious although the injury may not "look bad." Delayed damage may result from slow hemorrhage, injury to internal eye structures. Take no chances if eye has suffered a severe blunt blow. Have prompt examination by an eye physician. Important → Do not depend on first-aid measures alone. *Cold* compresses may be applied. Do *not* use hot compresses on eyes.

Foreign bodies in eye

It is safe to use simple first-aid measures to remove cinders, eyelashes, or specks which rest loosely on the surface of eyelid or eyeball. Do not attempt to remove imbedded particles that resist simple first-aid procedures. *Never rub or scratch* an eye that "has something in it." This may cause scars, or drive particles farther in. *Wash hands* before touching eyes.

Pull upper eyelid out and down over lower lid, or shut both eyes for a few minutes, to give flow of tears which may wash out the particle.

If this does not work, fill medicine dropper with warm water or boric acid solution, to "flood" eye and flush out foreign body.

If speck is visible (pull lower eyelid gently out and downward for

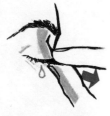

Keep upper eyelid pulled down several seconds; tears may remove particle

inspection) use *moistened* cotton applicator or corner of clean cotton cloth to lift out speck.

Do not use more vigorous methods to remove particles imbedded in lids or eyes. Cover with sterile gauze compress, held or gently taped in place. Get to doctor immediately.

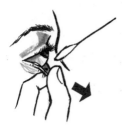

Remove speck with cotton applicator

Foreign bodies imbedded in eye

Penetrating eye wounds

All perforating wounds of the eye are serious, no matter how small, need *immediate medical help.* A tiny foreign body buried deep *inside* the eye may leave little outward trace. Do *not* apply oils or ointments. Cover *both* eyes with a sterile compress (to lessen harmful eye movements). Bandage *lightly* in place—no hard pressure. Get to doctor.

← Important

Transport victim flat on back on stretcher, if possible.

Some penetrating eye wounds, such as stabs from pointed objects, are obvious and terrifying, but some are not. A tiny piece of steel hurled off from tool grinding or pounding a nail may be lodged in an eye that "looks" normal. Anyone who has "felt something strike the eye" should be examined by a doctor promptly. Glass splinters, sand, transparent sharp particles, may not be visible to ordinary observation.

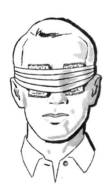

Apply loose bandage to eye; get medical aid immediately

eyes

Black eye

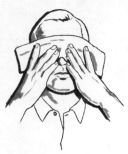

Hold a cold, wet compress against bruised eye

An "ordinary" black eye is a bruise. For *immediate* first aid, apply *pressure* to involved area, preferably with *cold* compresses or cloths wrung out of cold water. This helps to minimize discoloration *if done at once*. A doctor may inject an enzyme which promotes absorption of blood and disappearance of "black-and-blueness" at rapid rate. A severe black eye may involve deeper injury and need medical attention.

Prevent eye tragedies

Think of knives, scissors, needles, and pincushions as if they were deadly poisons to small children. Keep out of reach, off tables from which they may fall, be picked up or run into. Teach children never to play, run with or hurl sharp sticks or objects. Bows and arrows, BB guns, and unsafe toys should be kept from small children. Keep lye, cleansers, acids, household chemicals in a safe place; use carefully, never leave containers open. Hobbyists and do-it-yourselfers: caution with tools which may send metal or wood fragments flying. Wear protective goggles. Ordinary glasses give some protection. In industry, always wear protective goggles if provided.

Foreign bodies

Inhaled, swallowed, lodged in body orifices

Ear

Children may insert small objects into ear canal. Peas, beans, popcorn swell when wet, are hard to remove.

Do not dig at object with toothpick, hairpin, wire—grave danger of injuring ear canal or eardrum. You may push object further in.

Rarely is there any immediate danger. If object appears loose, gently pull ear lobe backwards and tilt child's head so object can fall out. If this fails, take patient to physician who has instruments to remove foreign body. If object is a bean or seed, a little olive oil or mineral oil can be dropped into ear to lessen swelling.

Insect in ear

If insect crawls into ear, turn head to one side and drop in some warm olive oil or mineral oil to suffocate insect. If no oil available, use warm water. Have physician remove insect.

Never try to remove foreign bodies lodged in ear or nose

Take to physician

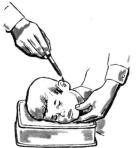

Suffocate insect with oil or warm water

foreign bodies

Eye

See *Eyes*, page 94

Nose

Children sometimes slip beans, grains and small objects into nose. No immediate danger, but great harm can be done trying to remove object with crude instruments. Drop olive oil into nostril to soothe tissues and prevent swelling. Patient may blow nose *gently*, never forcibly (*both* nostrils open) after oil is instilled. If this does not dislodge object, take to doctor.

Stomach

Tacks, open safety pins, needles and other small sharp objects are frequently swallowed by children. *Do not* give a laxative. May give child mashed potatoes. Take to doctor. Most foreign objects that reach the stomach pass through the bowel harmlessly, but the doctor may follow progress with a fluoroscope and use other measures. *Never* force a child who has swallowed a sharp object to vomit.

Throat, windpipe

See *choking*, page 14

Prevent foreign body accidents

Never give popcorn, candy, nuts, of cookies that contain nuts to small children who can't chew them and may inhale them. Don't let small children play with dry beans, peas, buttons, coins, nails, screws. Check stuffed animals and other toys for easily removable small parts which child may remove and swallow or stuff into body openings. Make a habit of closing safety pins every time you use them. Don't hold tacks, pins or nails in your mouth while doing chores, or let children see you doing so. Be sure that all bone fragments are removed from foods of small children.

Don't let small children play with objects they might swallow

Freezing injuries

Frostbite

Parts of body frozen, white or grayish-yellow, numb. Extremities and face most often frozen.

Do not rub frozen part with snow or anything else. Frozen tissue is fragile, easily damaged.

Do not expose frozen part to intense direct heat of hot stove, radiator, heat lamp.

If outdoors, thaw part by using patient's body or body of another as a warmer—frozen hand under armpit, between thighs; warm hand over frozen ear, nose.

In shelter, immerse frozen part in tepid (not hot) water, temperature about 100 degrees. Or, cover part with warmed—not hot—towels or blankets. See doctor for aftercare. If deeply frozen, serious, get doctor immediately.

Prolonged exposure to cold

Chilling of entire body, in degree from mild chilling to numbness, drowsiness, unconsciousness, and death unless rescued.

For mild chill, put patient to

Do not rub!
Frozen areas bruise easily; rubbing may result in gangrene

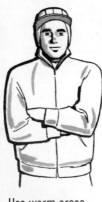

Use warm areas of the body to thaw frozen parts

bed in a warm room, cover well, give hot drinks.

For serious freezing exposure: Get victim to warm place. If breathing is imperceptible or stopped, give *artificial respiration.*

Rewarm rapidly by immersing in tub of water, 78 to 82 degrees.

Wrap victim in warm blankets; put him to bed.

Give warm drinks.

Get medical help.

100 degrees

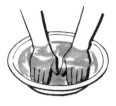

Immerse frozen part in warm water, or wrap in warm cloth

Heat illnesses

Heatstroke, sunstroke

Serious → Grave emergency. Often fatal. Act quickly to cool victim.

Symptoms: Very hot, absolutely dry skin, no sweating. Body temperature very high, 104 up to an incredible 110 degrees. Weakness, dizziness, rapid breathing, nausea, unconsciousness, sometimes mental confusion. Onset is often dramatically sudden.

Important → *Cool victim rapidly.* Apply ice bag, crushed ice in cloth, or cold cloths to head. If he can't be moved to shelter, drench his clothes with cold water, poured on or sprayed from hose.

Preferably, strip clothing, wrap him in sheet, keep sheet wet with cold water, place electric fans to blow on cold sheet. Keep cold cloths or ice on head.

At same time, *rub his arms and legs* toward the heart through sheet. Continue; important.

Massage arms and legs while patient cools

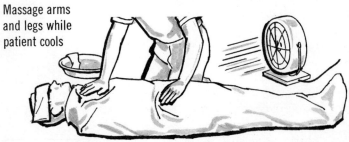

Check body temperature every 10 minutes or so, preferably by thermometer, or if necessary by feeling skin.

Keep repeating the cooling procedures until temperature drops to between 101 and 102 degrees. If temperature rises again, repeat cooling procedures.

Summon doctor immediately. ← Important

Heat exhaustion

Patient's skin is pallid, clammy, moist; profuse sweating. Temperature about normal, perhaps slightly lowered or slightly elevated. Nausea likely; scant urine; dizziness. Patient may faint.

Remove patient to circulating air; have him lie down, rest. Loosen clothing. Give sips of slightly salted water (1 teaspoonful of salt to pint). Stimulants: coffee, tea.

If symptoms do not pass away readily, call physician.

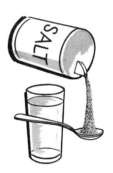
Give sips of salt water to victim

Heat cramps

Painful spasms of abdominal, leg or arm muscles. Caused by loss of body salt through profuse, prolonged sweating. Most common in persons who do very hard physical labor in extremely hot surroundings for long periods. Cramps usually respond to firm hand pressure, warm wet towels, hot water bottle. Give sips of slightly salted water.

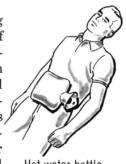
Hot water bottle may lessen cramps

Unconsciousness

Unconsciousness has many causes. If cause is known, or apparent from quick inspection, treat for Common causes → the particular emergency: *Sunstroke, poisoning, drowning, choking, electric shock, gas inhalation, concussion, fracture* are common causes.

If cause is not obvious, look quickly for clues: empty bottles, signs of blow, fall or accident, live wires, lip burns (corrosive poison).

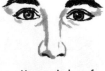

Unequal size of pupils is a sign of brain injury

Unequal pupils indicate brain injury or skull fracture (page 38). *Summon doctor immediately.* Do not assume that victim is drunk even though alcohol or other odors are detected. Look in victim's bag or wallet for card which may say he is a diabetic or subject to other emergencies. Do *not* shake an unconscious person to wake him up.

Important → *Never* try to give anything by mouth to an unconscious person.

Often a first-aider cannot determine the exact cause of unconsciousness.

What to do first
if patient is unconscious:

If breathing is inadequate or stopped, start artificial respiration at once.

If breathing is adequate, keep patient lying flat on back, warm but not hot, loosen constricting clothing, look for an apparent cause of unconsciousness such as a blow or fall. If the cause is obvious give proper first aid for that condition.

Summon physician, unless unconsciousness is very brief, as in common fainting. A person who has suffered a concussion or brief "knockout" should be seen by doctor even though recovery of consciousness is prompt.

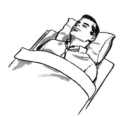

Keep victim flat on back; loosen collar and belt

Apoplexy (*Stroke*)

Caused by break or seepage from blood vessels within skull—usually in persons over 50 years of age.

Face red, but sometimes pale gray. Strong slow pulse. One eye pupil often larger than the other. One side of body or one limb may be limp, paralyzed; one corner of mouth may droop.

Keep patient quiet, warm but not hot. Apply cold cloths to head. Summon physician immediately. Transport patient in lying position if he must be moved.

Give no stimulants to apoplexy victim

Fainting

Most common form of pallid unconsciousness, caused by temporary insufficiency of blood supply to brain. Correct by getting head level with or lower than body.

If you feel faint, about to "pass out," lie down if possible. If not,

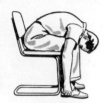

Lie down, sit, or
kneel at first
sign of faintness

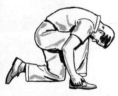

Keep head lowered
and breathe deeply

bend forward at waist from sitting position and put head between knees. If you can't lie or sit, kneel on one knee as if tying shoe, to get head lower than the heart.

In a crowded place, if someone feels faint, don't try to walk him out. Bend his head forward between knees until he feels better. Best first aid for fainting: Keep patient lying down, head lowered or legs and hips elevated. Cold water sprinkled on the face helps to stimulate recovery.

After consciousness is regained, coffee, tea may be given. Recovery should be rapid—five minutes or less. If unconsciousness is prolonged, or fainting fits recur, see physician.

Civil defense

Emergency measures

Prepare now to protect your family in the event of enemy nuclear attack. The following measures of protection are recommended by the Office of Defense and Civilian Mobilization.

Home shelter

Build an underground shelter, or select safest area in your home, preferably a basement corner, for use as emergency shelter.

Store these items in shelter:

Keep a two-week supply of food and water in your shelter. Rotate foods for kitchen use so emergency supply is kept fresh. Replace bottled water every three months. Store a battery radio, flashlight, blankets and warm clothing, a first-aid kit containing water purification tablets and toilet soap. Store items so a three-day supply can be transferred quickly to your car.

Warning signals

Civil defense warning devices may be sirens, horns, or whistles.
There are two distinct signals

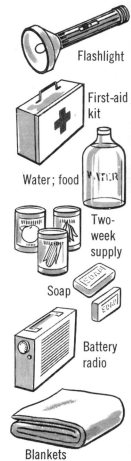

Emergency items

Flashlight

First-aid kit

Water; food

Two-week supply

Soap

Battery radio

Blankets

Tune radio to
640 or **1240**
for official information

for public action directed by local government:

1. *A long steady blast* of 3 to 5 minutes duration means alert. Attack may come soon. Tune your radio dial to 640 or 1240—frequencies of Conelrad stations which will broadcast official information. Take action as directed by your local community. Do not attempt to use telephone.

2. A three-minute warbling tone or series of short blasts means take cover. *Attack is imminent.* Take cover immediately in best available shelter.

If in a building without a prepared shelter, go to basement or interior room on first floor.

If outdoors or in a car, go to nearest shelter—if you cannot, lie face down on ground or crouch on floor of the car.

When directed to take shelter or evacuate your home or office:

Close all doors and windows; draw blinds.

Turn off all electricity at main switch, or disconnect all electrical appliances.

Turn off gas range burners or room heaters.

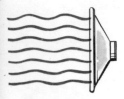

Steady blast, 3 to 5 minutes long—alert

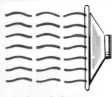

Series of short blasts—take cover

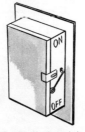

Turn off electricity

Fallout protection

Any protection against radioactive particles is better than none. An underground shelter, covered with at least three feet of earth and properly ventilated, is safest. An ordinary basement with windows and entryways sandbagged will give some protection. If nothing better, a frame house will reduce the danger, especially if you stay on the lowest floor near the center.

Decontamination

Go to center of lowest floor in a frame house

Radioactive fallout, like dust, can be removed from most surfaces by washing, vacuum cleaning, plowing under. Danger increases with length of exposure. *Except* for immediate personal de- ← Important
contamination, such as removal of contaminated outer garments, decontamination should be carried out only under official instructions of local authorities who will tell you what you should do and how much time you have to do it.

Know your community's plan for emergency action. Your city or county government officials will inform you. If no local plan exists, get in touch with Civil Defense Headquarters of your state government for co-operation with local officials in setting up a program. At least one member of the family should take a Red Cross course in first aid. Keep a copy of this first-aid book with supplies in your home shelter.

Personal health log

Your family doctor keeps your health record in his files. But during a lifetime you may move to new places, consult new doctors. Records may be lost; memory is unreliable. A permanent record in your possession is of great value when it is desirable to know exact dates, past illnesses, treatments and who gave them, and other important facts. Keep a permanent personal health log for each member of the family, with help of your doctor who knows what information is important. *Date* all entries. Give the name and address of each *doctor* who has given treatment and who keeps the full medical record.

Vaccinations need to be renewed periodically

Immunizing "shots" do not last a lifetime. Ask your doctor if your vaccinations are "wearing out." Some vaccines are needed only in special circumstances; the vaccines and booster shots listed in the chart below are of universal importance:

VACCINE	PROTECTION
Smallpox Needed by everyone.	3 to 7 years, sometimes longer. For maximum protection, re-vaccination every 3 years.
Polio (Salk-type vaccine) Needed by everyone under 40 years of age and recommended for all ages.	Uncertain. Booster dose desirable one year after primary immunization.
Diphtheria, Whooping Cough, Tetanus (4-way vaccines include polio) Combined vaccines, for all babies.	Booster for tetanus (and diphtheria, if doctor recommends) every 3 years up to age 15.
Influenza If doctor recommends.	Probably 8 months or more —repeat yearly.

Get vaccinations before traveling abroad

You will need certain vaccinations to enter foreign countries and re-enter the United States. Requirements vary according to places you visit. Documents and information are available from the clerk of the Federal Court in your district, from Department of State passport agencies, and from travel agencies, ticket offices, local and state health departments, and offices of the United States Public Health Service.

Name_____

Blood type_____Rh factor_____

Vaccinations_____Date_____

_____

Booster_____

Blood transfusions_____

X rays_____

_____

Hospitals entered_____

Laboratory findings_____

Significant illnesses_____

_____

_____

_____

Surgical operations_____

_____

_____

Drug sensitivities, allergies_____

_____

_____

Other information by M.D._____

_____

_____

_____

_____

Name_____

Blood type_____ Rh factor_____

Vaccinations_____ Date_____

_____

_____

Booster_____

Blood transfusions_____

X rays_____

_____

Hospitals entered_____

Laboratory findings_____

Significant illnesses_____

_____

_____

_____

Surgical operations_____

_____

_____

_____

Drug sensitivities, allergies_____

_____

_____

Other information by M.D._____

_____

_____

_____

_____

Name_____

Blood type_____Rh factor_____

Vaccinations_____Date_____

_____

Booster_____

Blood transfusions_____

X rays_____

_____

Hospitals entered_____

Laboratory findings_____

Significant illnesses_____

_____

_____

_____

_____

Surgical operations_____

_____

_____

_____

Drug sensitivities, allergies_____

_____

_____

Other information by M.D._____

_____

_____

_____

_____

Name_____

Blood type_____Rh factor_____

Vaccinations_____Date_____

Booster_____

Blood transfusions_____

X rays_____

Hospitals entered_____

Laboratory findings_____

Significant illnesses_____

_____

_____

_____

Surgical operations_____

_____

_____

_____

Drug sensitivities, allergies_____

_____

_____

Other information by M.D._____

_____

_____

_____

_____

Name_____

Blood type_____Rh factor_____

Vaccinations_____Date_____

Booster_____

Blood transfusions_____

X rays_____

Hospitals entered_____

Laboratory findings_____

Significant illnesses_____

Surgical operations_____

Drug sensitivities, allergies_____

Other information by M.D._____

Name_____

Blood type_____Rh factor_____

Vaccinations_____Date_____

_____

Booster_____

Blood transfusions_____

X rays_____

_____

Hospitals entered_____

Laboratory findings_____

Significant illnesses_____

_____

_____

_____

Surgical operations_____

_____

_____

_____

Drug sensitivities, allergies_____

_____

_____

Other information by M.D._____

_____

_____

_____

Name_____

Blood type_____Rh factor____

Vaccinations_____Date____

_____

Booster_____

Blood transfusions_____

X rays_____

_____

Hospitals entered_____

Laboratory findings_____

Significant illnesses_____

_____

_____

_____

_____

Surgical operations_____

_____

_____

_____

Drug sensitivities, allergies_____

_____

_____

Other information by M.D._____

_____

_____

_____

_____

_____

Index